Comparative-Effectiveness Research in Heart Failure

Editor

MARK HLATKY

HEART FAILURE CLINICS

www.heartfailure.theclinics.com

Founding Editor
JAGAT NARULA

January 2013 • Volume 9 • Number 1

ELSEVIER

1600 John F. Kennedy Boulevard • Suite 1800 • Philadelphia, Pennsylvania 19103-2899

http://www.theclinics.com

HEART FAILURE CLINICS Volume 9, Number 1
January 2013 ISSN 1551-7136, ISBN-13: 978-1-4557-7098-4

Editor: Barbara Cohen-Kligerman

Heart Failure Clinics (ISSN 1551-7136) is published quarterly by Elsevier Inc., 360 Park Avenue South, New York, NY 10010-1710. Months of publication are January, April, July, and October. Business and editorial offices: 1600 John F. Kennedy Boulevard, Suite 1800, Philadelphia, PA 19103-2899. Periodicals postage paid at New York, NY, and additional mailing offices. Subscription prices are USD 224.00 per year for US individuals, USD 361.00 per year for US institutions, USD 76.00 per year for US students and residents, USD 268.00 per year for Canadian individuals, USD 413.00 per year for Canadian institutions, USD 285.00 per year for international individuals, USD 413.00 per year for international institutions, and USD 96.00 per year for Canadian and foreign students/residents. To receive student and resident rate, orders must be accompanied by name of affiliated institution, date of term, and the *signature* of program/residency coordinator on institution letterhead. Orders will be billed at individual rate until proof of status is received. Foreign air speed delivery is included in all *Clinics* subscription prices. All prices are subject to change without notice. **POSTMASTER:** Send address changes to *Heart Failure Clinics*, Elsevier Health Sciences Division, Subscription Customer Service, 3251 Riverport Lane, Maryland Heights, MO 63043. **Customer Service: 1-800-654-2452 (US and Canada). From outside of the US and Canada, call 314-447-8871. Fax: 314-447-8029. For print support, e-mail: JournalsCustomerService-usa@elsevier.com. For online support, e-mail: JournalsOnlineSupport-usa@elsevier.com.**

Reprints. For copies of 100 or more of articles in this publication, please contact the Commercial Reprints Department, Elsevier Inc., 360 Park Avenue South, New York, NY 10010-1710. Tel.: 212-633-3812; Fax: 212-462-1935; E-mail: reprints@elsevier.com.

Heart Failure Clinics is covered in *MEDLINE/PubMed (Index Medicus)*.

Printed and bound by CPI Group (UK) Ltd, Croydon, CR0 4YY

Transferred to digital print 2012

Contributors

GUEST EDITOR

MARK HLATKY, MD
Professor of Health Research and Policy;
Professor of Medicine (Cardiovascular
Medicine), Stanford University School of
Medicine, Stanford, California

AUTHORS

SUZANNE ADAMS, RN, MPH
Manager, Outcomes Research and Education,
Coordinating Center for Clinical Research,
Jefferson Medical College, Philadelphia,
Pennsylvania

LARRY A. ALLEN, MD, MHS
Assistant Professor of Medicine, Division of
Cardiology, University of Colorado School of
Medicine, Aurora, Colorado

TARA I. CHANG, MD, MS
Department of Medicine, Stanford University,
Palo Alto, California

PAUL S. COROTTO, MD
Resident, UPMC Internal Medicine, UPMC
Montefiore Hospital, University of Pittsburgh
Medical Center, Pittsburgh, Pennsylvania

LESLEY H. CURTIS, PhD
Duke Clinical Research Institute and
Department of Medicine, Duke University
School of Medicine, Durham, North Carolina

GREGG C. FONAROW, MD
Department of Medicine, University of
California, Los Angeles, Los Angeles, California

EMIL L. FOSBOL, MD, PhD
Duke Clinical Research Institute, Duke
University Medical Center, Durham,
North Carolina

JAMES V. FREEMAN, MD, MPH, MS
Division of Cardiovascular Medicine, Stanford
University School of Medicine, Stanford,
California

BRADLEY G. HAMMILL, MS
Duke Clinical Research Institute, Durham,
North Carolina

MARK HLATKY, MD
Professor of Health Research and Policy;
Professor of Medicine (Cardiovascular
Medicine), Stanford University School of
Medicine, Stanford, California

DHRUV S. KAZI, MD, MSc, MS
Assistant Adjunct Professor, Division of
Cardiology, Department of Medicine,
University of California, San Francisco,
San Francisco, California

PRATEETI KHAZANIE, MD, MPH
Cardiology Fellow, Duke University, Durham,
North Carolina

DANIEL B. MARK, MD, MPH
Director, Outcomes Research Group, Duke
Clinical Research Institute; Professor of
Medicine, Duke University Medical Center,
Durham, North Carolina

FREDERICK A. MASOUDI, MD, MSPH
Division of Cardiology, University of Colorado
Denver, Aurora, Colorado

MELISSA M. MCCAREY, BA
Research Assistant, Outcomes Research
and Education, Coordinating Center for
Clinical Research, Jefferson Medical College,
Philadelphia, Pennsylvania

SOKO SETOGUCHI, MD, DrPH
Associate Professor of Medicine, Duke
University Medical Center, Durham,
North Carolina

RASHMEE U. SHAH, MD, MS
Department of Cardiology, Cedars-Sinai
Medical Center, Stanford University, Stanford,
California

JOHN A. SPERTUS, MD, MPH
Professor of Medicine, Saint Luke's Mid
America Heart Institute, University of Missouri,
Kansas City, Missouri

DAVID J. WHELLAN, MD, MHS
Associate Professor, Director, Coordinating
Center for Clinical Research, Jefferson Medical
College, Philadelphia, Pennsylvania

**WOLFGANG C. WINKELMAYER, MD,
MPH, ScD**
Associate Professor of Medicine, Stanford
University, Stanford, California

YING XIAN, MD, PhD
Duke Clinical Research Institute and
Department of Medicine, Duke University
School of Medicine, Durham, North Carolina

Contents

HEART FAILURE CLINICS

DOWNLOAD Free App!

Review Articles THE CLINICS

NOW AVAILABLE FOR YOUR iPhone and iPad

Preface
Comparative Effectiveness Research in Heart Failure

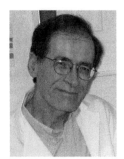

Mark Hlatky, MD
Guest Editor

Comparative effectiveness research has emerged as a new and important field, fostered by recent efforts to reform the health care system, and by the creation of the Patient-Centered Outcomes Research Institute. Comparative effectiveness research aims to provide reliable evidence about the effectiveness and safety of clinical management strategies, with a particular emphasis on "real-world" practices and outcomes. Comparative effectiveness research has a greater focus on documenting what works in practice and how well alternative treatments compare with each other, rather than with a placebo.

This issue of the *Heart Failure Clinics* contains a series of articles that examines the application of comparative effectiveness research to heart failure. My associates, Alan Go and Adrian Hernandez, and I selected several articles that review the methods and data sources used in comparative effectiveness research, and several articles that examine specific applications of these methods to the management of patients with heart failure. We believe that you will find these articles to be a concise and rigorous review of comparative effectiveness research in heart failure.

Mark Hlatky, MD
Stanford University School of Medicine
HRP Redwood Building, Room 150
Stanford, CA 94305-5405, USA

E-mail address:
hlatky@stanford.edu

http://dx.doi.org/10.1016/j.hfc.2012.09.009
1551-7136/13/$ – see front matter

heartfailure.theclinics.com

Data Sources for Heart Failure Comparative Effectiveness Research

Ying Xian, MD, PhD[a,b], Bradley G. Hammill, MS[a],
Lesley H. Curtis, PhD[a,b],*

KEYWORDS

- Comparative effectiveness research • Heart failure research • Clinical registries • Databases

KEY POINTS

- Existing data sources for heart failure research offer advantages and disadvantages for comparative effectiveness research.
- Clinical registries collect detailed information about disease presentation, treatment, and outcomes on a large number of patients and provide the "real-world" population that is the hallmark of comparative effectiveness research. Data are not collected longitudinally, however, and follow-up is often limited.
- Large administrative datasets provide the broadest population coverage with longitudinal outcomes follow-up but lack clinical detail.
- Linking clinical registries with other databases to assess longitudinal outcomes holds great promise.

Heart failure is one of the major public health problems in the United States, affecting 5.8 million Americans and costing $39.2 billion in 2010.[1] Despite significant advances in the diagnosis and management of patients with heart failure, the comparative effectiveness of these treatments and strategies in "real world" settings remains unclear. According to the Federal Coordinating Council for Comparative Effectiveness Research, the purpose of comparative effectiveness research (CER) is to assist clinicians and patients in making informed health care decisions and to improve the health of communities and the performance of the health system.[2] CER can take many forms including randomized controlled trials (RCTs), systematic reviews of the literature, and observational studies using clinical registries, administrative data, and electronic medical records. Indeed, the council expressed its support for efforts that "encourage the development and use of clinical registries, clinical data networks, and other forms of electronic health data that can be used to generate or obtain outcomes data."[3] We review existing data sources for CER in heart failure, examine their strengths and limitations, and identify potential opportunities for further development.

GENERAL DATA NEEDS FOR CER

High-quality CER is critically dependent on the reliability and robustness of the underlying data. Several characteristics of the data sources must be considered, including the relevance of the study population, the validity of exposure (treatment) and outcome (effectiveness) measurements, and the ability to control for confounders.

Unlike an RCT that compares the efficacy of different medications under ideal conditions in

[a] Duke Clinical Research Institute, Duke University School of Medicine, PO Box 17969, Durham, NC, USA;
[b] Department of Medicine, Duke University School of Medicine, Box 3230 Medical Center, Durham, NC 27710, Durham, NC, USA
* Corresponding author. Duke Clinical Research Institute, PO Box 17969, Durham, NC 27715.
E-mail address: lesley.curtis@duke.edu

Heart Failure Clin 9 (2013) 1–13
http://dx.doi.org/10.1016/j.hfc.2012.09.001
1551-7136/13/$ – see front matter © 2013 Elsevier Inc. All rights reserved.

carefully selected patients, CER aims to estimate the effectiveness of treatments or strategies as they are used in "real world" settings.[2] Data sources for CER, therefore, should represent the broad population and include patient populations typically underrepresented in clinical trials. Indeed, the Federal Coordinating Council for Comparative Effectiveness Research emphasized the inclusion of racial/ethnic minorities, children, elderly, individuals with multiple chronic conditions, and those with disabilities in CER.[2]

In addition, data sources for CER must include information regarding exposures, outcomes, and potential confounders. The definition and measurement of these elements should be clear. When evaluating the adequacy of some exposure, outcome, or confounder for a study, the precision or accuracy of the measure in capturing the concept of interest should be considered. The scale of the measurement, whether continuous or categorical, and the period of time during which a measurement is ascertained should also be considered. For example, if using receipt of β-blockers as an exposure, how much detail is available about receipt of that medication by a study subject? Did the subject receive a prescription for the medication? Did he fill the prescription? Did he ingest the medication? Do we have longitudinal information about dose and medication supply? And what time period of prior exposure is available and relevant? If using mortality or readmission as an outcome, is it possible to know the cause of the event? And was long-term follow-up available, or are we limited to events proximate to the exposure? If using hypertension as a potential confounder, do we only have an indicator for presence of the comorbidity? If so, how was that indicator defined? And was it based on medical records or patient self-report? Do we instead have continuous blood pressure data available?

CLINICAL REGISTRIES

Like RCTs, clinical registries typically rely on prospective data collection according to a well-defined protocol with standardized data definitions. Importantly, however, clinical registries record the treatment that is administered and do not constrain treatment assignment. In this section, we begin by reviewing 3 major heart failure registries, highlighting their history and selected scientific contributions (**Table 1**). Next, we briefly describe other registries that, although not limited to the heart failure population, include a substantial proportion of patients with heart failure (**Table 2**). Finally, we summarize the strengths and limitations of clinical registries for CER.

Heart Failure Registries

The Organized Program to Initiate Life-Saving Treatment in Hospitalized patients with Heart Failure (OPTIMIZE-HF) registry is a national registry designed to evaluate and improve guideline adherence among hospitalized patients with heart failure.[4] Patients hospitalized for worsening heart failure or those in whom significant heart failure symptoms developed during hospitalization were eligible. Participating hospitals (N = 259) enrolled more than 50,000 patients from January 1, 2003, through December 31, 2004. In addition to detailed clinical data, information regarding in-hospital interventions, medications at discharge, and in-hospital outcomes were collected. In a sample of patients, outcome data were obtained at 60 and 90 days following discharge. Initially supported by GlaxoSmithKline, administration of the OPTIMIZE-HF program was transitioned to the American Heart Association (AHA) in 2005 as part of the Get with the Guidelines (GWTG) program, and OPTIMIZE-HF data are included in the GWTG–Heart Failure (GWTG-HF) registry.

The registry has been used extensively to describe patients hospitalized for heart failure[5–11] and the care they receive[12–14] and to examine the association between care and outcomes.[15–19] In one analysis, researchers examined the association between adherence to practice guidelines for the diagnosis and management of chronic heart failure and subsequent outcomes.[19] The authors identified 5791 patients with heart failure hospitalized at 91 hospitals in the OPTIMIZE-HF registry. Using propensity score analysis accounting for potential confounders that related to performance measure selection bias, the results suggested that adherence to angiotensin-converting enzyme inhibitor or angiotensin receptor blocker and β-blocker at discharge was associated with reduced mortality and combined mortality/hospitalization within 90 days following discharge. More recently, OPTIMIZE-HF data were used to examine the association between initiation of β-blocker therapy at discharge and long-term outcomes.[17] Investigators linked the registry with Medicare claims data to obtain long-term follow-up and found that initiation of β-blocker therapy was clinically effective and independently associated with lower risks of rehospitalization and death.

The AHA GWTG-HF is a continuous quality improvement program funded by the AHA that focuses on the redesign of hospitals' systems of care to improve the quality of care received by patients with heart failure.[20] GWTG-HF uses a Web-based Patient Management Tool (Outcomes, Cambridge, MA) to abstract detailed clinical data

Table 1
Heart failure registries

Registry	Population	Exposure	Outcomes	Confounder/Clinical Variables
OPTIMIZE-HF	~50,000 Patients with heart failure at 259 academic and community hospitals in the United States	Medication, in-hospital care and intervention	The Joint Commission performance measurements, in-hospital clinical events and mortality. 60- and 90-day outcomes for a small subset of patients. Can be linked to external datasets for long-term outcomes using indirect identifiers.	Patient demographic, detailed medical history, vital signs, laboratory information, diagnosis, medications, in-hospital care and interventions
GWTG-HF	~530,000 HF patients at 558 academic and community hospitals in the United States	Medication, in-hospital care and intervention	GWTG-HF quality measures, in-hospital clinical events and mortality. Can be linked to external datasets for long-term outcomes using indirect identifiers.	Patient demographic, detailed medical history, vital signs, laboratory information, diagnosis, medications, in-hospital care and interventions.
ADHERE Registry	~150,000 Patients with heart failure in >300 academic and community hospitals in the United States	Medication, in-hospital care and intervention	The Joint Commission performance measurements, in-hospital clinical events, and mortality. Can be linked to external datasets for long-term outcomes using indirect identifiers.	Patient demographic, detailed medical history, vital signs, laboratory information, diagnosis, medications, in-hospital care and interventions.

Table 2
Other cardiovascular registries

Registry	Population	Exposure	Outcomes	Confounder/Clinical Variables
NCDR ICD Registry	~380,000 ICD implants with 88% of New York Heart Association functional class II–IV	ICD implantation, device type, procedure characteristics, and medication	Compliance with the ACC/AHA/HRS clinical guidelines recommendations, intraprocedural/postprocedural clinical event and mortality. Direct identifier (name, date of birth, Social Security number) are collected to enable linkage to National Death Index and other administrative databases (eg, Medicare 100% fee-for-service (FFS) inpatient claims) to conduct longitudinal follow-up	Patient demographic, medical history, baseline tests, ICD indication, ICD type, in-hospital care, in-hospital adverse events
NCDR Action Registry-GWTG	~150,000 Patients with coronary artery disease; 12%, of whom have previous medical history of heart failure and 7% have new or recurrent heart failure.	Medication, in-hospital care and intervention	GWTG-HF quality measures, in-hospital clinical events and mortality. Direct identifier (name, date of birth, Social Security number) are collected to enable linkage with to National Death Index and other administrative databases to conduct longitudinal follow-up	Patient demographic, detailed medical history, vital signs, laboratory information, diagnosis, medication treatment, in-hospital care, and intervention. Zip code–level socioeconomic status by linking to external data sources
STS Adult Cardiac Surgery Database	~4.3 Million patients who underwent coronary artery bypass graft surgery, valve surgery, mechanical cardiac assist devices, or another cardiac procedure, 90% of whom are on New York Heart Association functional class II–IV	Cardiac surgery, procedure characteristics, medication	In-hospital clinical events, mortality, 30-day readmission. Direct identifier (name, date of birth, Social Security number) are collected to enable linkage with to National Death Index and other administrative databases (eg, Medicare 100% FFS inpatient claims) to conduct longitudinal follow-up	Patient demographic, clinical risk factors, previous cardiac interventions, perioperative cardiac status/medications, hemodynamics/Cath/Echo, detailed in-hospital procedure/intervention. Zip code–level socioeconomic status by linking with external data sources

including patient demographics, medical history, symptoms on arrival, in-hospital treatment and events, discharge treatment and counseling, and patient disposition. Data collection began in 2005 and continues with more than 500,000 records from 558 participating sites as of May 2011.

To date, the registry has been used to describe the quality of care[21-28] provided to patients hospitalized with heart failure and how that care differs by race and sex.[29-31] In addition, the GWTG-HF and OPTIMIZE-HF registries have been combined with Medicare claims data and used to generate evidence regarding the clinical effectiveness of implantable cardioverter-defibrillators (ICDs).[26] Of 4685 patients eligible for an ICD implant, 376 (8%) received an ICD before discharge. After adjustment, Medicare beneficiaries hospitalized with heart failure who were selected for ICD therapy had lower long-term mortality compared with those who were not selected for ICD therapy. More recently, the data were used to examine the relation between early physician follow-up after a hospitalization for heart failure and 30-day readmission.[32] The results suggested that patients who are discharged from hospitals that have higher rates of follow-up within 7 days of discharge have a lower risk of 30-day readmission.

The Acute Decompensated Heart Failure National Registry (ADHERE) is a large multicenter national registry to evaluate characteristics, management, and clinical outcomes among patients hospitalized with acute decompensated heart failure.[4] More than 150,000 patients from 300 community and academic centers in the United States were enrolled between September 2001 and March 2006. This industry-sponsored registry (by Scios Inc, Fremont, California) is rich with clinical detail (eg, cardiac troponin, B-type natriuretic peptide levels, and QRS duration) and includes information about the initial emergency department visit. Importantly, elderly patients enrolled in ADHERE are similar to Medicare beneficiaries hospitalized with heart failure, thereby supporting the generalizability of ADHERE-based studies.[3]

Similar to the other inpatient heart failure registries, ADHERE has been used extensively to describe the clinical characteristics of patients hospitalized with heart failure,[2,33-36] the association of those characteristics with outcomes,[37-40] and the relation between heart failure therapies and outcomes.[41-43] In one analysis, investigators examined the association between morphine and outcomes in 147,362 ADHERE patients, of whom 15% received morphine. After risk adjustment and exclusion of patients who required mechanical ventilation, morphine was strongly and independently associated with mortality.[42] Another analysis

compared the outcomes of patients who were initiated on nesiritide in the emergency department with outcomes of patients whose therapy was initiated in an inpatient unit.[41] Compared with patients initiated on therapy in an inpatient unit, patients initiated on therapy in the emergency department had shorter lengths of stay and were less likely to require transfer to the intensive care unit.

Other Cardiovascular Registries

Because of the high prevalence of heart failure, registries focused on other cardiovascular conditions may also be useful in performing CER. The American College of Cardiology (ACC)'s National Cardiovascular Data Registry for Implantable Cardioverter Defibrillators (NCDR-ICD) was launched in 2005 by the ACC and the Heart Rhythm Society in response to a mandate from the Centers for Medicare and Medicaid Services (CMS).[44] As of 2008, nearly 1500 hospitals participated in the NCDR-ICD registry and have contributed data for more than 380,000 implantations in the United States. Although data collection is mandatory only for Medicare beneficiaries, 88% of the participating hospitals submit data for all ICD implantations.[45] More than 130 data elements are collected at the time of the procedure, including patient demographics, clinical characteristics, device type, procedure, outcomes, and hospital performance data. The vast majority (74%) of patients have a history of heart failure.[46]

The ACC Acute Coronary Treatment and Intervention Outcomes Network (ACTION) was established through a series of mergers between the National Registry of Myocardial Infarction (NRMI) and the Can Rapid Risk Stratification of Unstable Angina Patients Suppress Adverse Outcomes with Early Implementation of the ACC/AHA Guidelines (CRUSADE) Registry in January 2007 and with the AHA GWTG–Coronary Artery Disease Program in June 2008.[47] The resulting NCDR–ACTION Registry–GWTG is the largest national quality improvement initiative focused on high-risk patients with myocardial infarction, collecting detailed demographic, clinical, process of care, and in-hospital outcomes data. Data from the older registries have been pooled and are included in the NCDR–ACTION Registry–GWTG. Information on heart failure is collected as a component of past medical history, at the time of first medical contact, and as an in-hospital clinical event. From 2007 to 2010, the NCDR–ACTION Registry–GWTG collected nearly 150,000 records from 383 participating hospitals in the United States.[11] Among those, 12% had a medical history of congestive heart failure and 7% had in-hospital clinical event of either new-onset or acute reoccurrence of heart failure.[47,48]

The Society of Thoracic Surgeons (STS) Adult Cardiac Surgery Database was established in June 1990 and is now the largest cardiothoracic surgery quality improvement and outcomes databases in the world.[49,50] The STS provides clinical details and outcomes for 4.3 million coronary artery bypass graft surgery, valve replacement and repair, and other cardiac procedures from 1014 participating sites, which represent 94% of adult cardiac centers in the United States. Data elements include patient demographics, clinical risk factors, previous cardiac interventions, preoperative cardiac status and medication, operative details, and postoperative events and outcomes. Heart failure is collected in the context of previous medical history, and New York Heart Association functional class is collected preoperatively. Among patients who underwent valve surgery or coronary artery bypass graft surgery, nearly 190,000 had a medical history of heart failure.[51–53]

Strengths and Limitations of Clinical Registries

Clinical registries have many strengths, including their size, broad population coverage, and well-defined measures of exposures and outcomes. Additionally, registries often include rich clinical information about risk factors and comorbidities to facilitate confounder adjustment. Importantly, compared with the selective enrollment and structured protocols of RCTs, clinical registries may better reflect how care is delivered in clinical practice. As a result, registries can support the evaluation of the effectiveness of interventions in which randomization is unethical or impractical.

Registry participation is usually voluntary, however, and the institutions that choose to participate may differ from those that do not. Therefore, the representativeness of patients enrolled in registries cannot be taken for granted and should be assessed on a case-by-case basis. Most registries enroll patients during a hospitalization and hence do not capture patients with heart failure who were diagnosed and treated as outpatients. Furthermore, many registries collect data only during a hospital admission and have no data on postdischarge care and long-term outcomes. Although methods have been developed to link clinical registries with external data sources (see later in this article), the cross-sectional data captured during a single inpatient stay may be less relevant to many questions of interest in CER. Finally, registries that are device- or procedure-based typically capture data only on patients who receive the device or undergo the procedure. Comparisons with eligible but unexposed patients require the addition of an external data source.

RCT DATABASES

RCT databases have many of the necessary attributes of a reliable and robust database for CER. Exposures are carefully defined, outcomes are objectively measured, and clinical characteristics are captured in detail. Despite having clinically rich data, RCT databases are not ideal for CER. RCTs are designed to evaluate the efficacy and safety of a treatment or intervention under ideal circumstances, which may differ substantially from the circumstances under which the treatment is used in clinical practice. In addition, RCT populations are usually narrowly selected,[54,55] so RCT databases may not represent the patients who will eventually receive the treatment in clinical practice. The essence of CER is to assess effectiveness in a "real-world" setting; on this count, RCT databases fall short.

Despite the limitations, RCT databases may find their way into observational CER. For example, the placebo arm of a device trial could potentially be used as the comparator for a device registry. As noted earlier, the registry population is likely to be representative of patients who receive devices, whereas the trial population is likely to be narrowly selected. Although the RCT database may have all of the data necessary for a comparison, the comparability of the 2 populations is questionable. An RCT database might also be used to examine outcomes associated with an other-than-randomized treatment. For example, a heart failure trial examining the efficacy of one therapy could be used as the database for an observational study of outcomes associated with another therapy for which data were collected. The richness of the data source notwithstanding, the analysis would provide little information regarding the effectiveness of the treatment as used in "real world" settings.

ADMINISTRATIVE DATA

Administrative data are electronic data that are typically generated and gathered for some administrative purpose, typically billing a payer for the provision of health services. These data can also be used for clinical research because they usually include patient demographics, disease diagnoses, and procedures received and sometimes include medications dispensed. There is increasing interest in using large administrative data for CER. Among all data sources discussed earlier, administrative data perhaps have the broadest population coverage, an attribute especially appealing to CERs. For example, Medicare provided health care to more than 43 million people in 2006, including 36 million beneficiaries who were aged 65 years and older.[56] **Table 3** lists common sources of administrative data.

Medicare and Medicaid Data

The Medicare health insurance program covers most Americans 65 years of age and older, in addition to certain younger individuals with disabilities or kidney failure. As of 2008, Medicare covered more than 45 million individuals.[57] CMS makes Medicare and Medicaid claims data available for research. Medicare data include claims for payment filed by institutional and noninstitutional providers, such as inpatient facilities, outpatient facilities, short-term skilled nursing facilities, hospice facilities and agencies, home health agencies, physicians, and durable medical equipment providers. As of 2006, CMS also makes available data on prescription medications dispensed. In addition to payments made by Medicare to providers, these claims contain information about diagnoses, procedures, and other health care utilization but do not contain laboratory test results. Medicare also provides a denominator file that includes demographic data, residence information, date of death, if applicable, and program eligibility and enrollment information for all beneficiaries. Beneficiaries can be identified in both the claims and denominator files with a unique identifier that allows for the creation of a longitudinal claims history. Medicare data are made available for a 5% sample of all Medicare beneficiaries, but data for 100% of a defined cohort can be requested. The 100% inpatient claims data are also made available for research by CMS in a format called the Medicare Provider Analysis and Review (MedPAR) file.[58]

Medicaid is a state-administered benefit that provides health insurance for individuals in federally mandated eligibility groups with limited income including children, pregnant women, disabled, and the elderly.[59] Specific benefits vary by state. The Medicaid Analytic eXtract formerly known as State Medicaid Research Files is a set of person-level data files containing information on Medicaid beneficiaries' eligibility, enrollment status, demographics, and utilization, including inpatient care, long-term care, medication claims, and claims for all noninstitutional Medicaid services.[60] These files are not available nationally but instead are state specific.

Recently, Medicare and Medicaid claims data were used to estimate the comparative effectiveness of β-blocker therapy in elderly patients with heart failure. The study population included 11,959 North Carolina residents aged 65 years and older who were eligible for Medicare and Medicaid and hospitalized for heart failure from 2001 through 2004. Evidence-based β-blockers (carvedilol, metoprolol succinate, and bisoprolol fumarate) were compared with non–evidence-based β-blockers with respect to survival, rehospitalization, and outpatient visits. After adjustment, the comparative effectiveness of evidence-based and non–evidence-based β-blockers was similar for 1-year survival but the rehospitalization rate was higher among patients who received evidence-based β-blockers.[61]

Veterans Health Administration Datasets

In 2010, more than 22.7 million individuals were enrolled to receive health care benefits and services from the Veterans Health Administration (VHA).[62] Data about their utilization are available in several files. The Patient Treatment File contains records on all inpatient care and includes diagnosis, procedure, and summary information on each episode of care. The Outpatient Clinic File contains records on all outpatient care. The Pharmacy Benefits Management Services Database contains all prescription dispensed within the VHA system from 1999 to present. And the Decision Support System Data Extracts contain cost and utilization information on inpatient and outpatient laboratory tests, pharmacy prescriptions, and radiologic procedures. Unlike other administrative data, laboratory test results for a specific list of tests are included in the Decision Support System. Like the Medicare denominator file, the Vital Status File contains demographic data, eligibility and enrollment information, and date of death information for all veterans who have received Veterans Administration care or benefits.[63]

Using VHA data, Desai[64] estimated the comparative effectiveness of angiotensin receptor blockers on the risk of mortality in 1536 patients diagnosed with chronic heart failure from October 1996 through September 2002. After adjustment for measured confounders, losartan, candesartan, irbesartan, and valsartan were found to be similarly effective in reducing survival.

Other Administrative Data Sources

The Health Care Cost and Utilization Project, which is sponsored by the Agency for Healthcare Research and Quality, includes the largest collection of longitudinal hospital care data in the United States.[65] The Health Care Cost and Utilization Project includes Nationwide Inpatient Sample (NIS) and State Inpatient Databases (SID). The NIS

Table 3
Administrative data

Database	Population	Clinical Variables	Health Outcomes	Laboratory Information	Medication Information
Medicare claims data	Medicare beneficiaries	Inpatient and outpatient diagnosis and procedures	Utilization and costs, mortality, longitudinal follow-up	No	Yes, for beneficiaries enrolled in Part D
Medicaid claims data (MAX)	Medicaid population	Inpatient, long-term care diagnoses and procedures. Only Medicaid covered services (coverage varies by state)	Service utilization and payments. Link to Medicare to identify dually eligible beneficiaries.	No	Yes
VA	Veterans of the US military	Inpatient and outpatient diagnoses and procedures	Cost and utilization, mortality, longitudinal follow-up	Yes	Yes
HCUP	All-payer inpatient care database NIS: 5–8 million inpatient stays from ~1000 hospitals each year. SID: 90% of all US community hospital discharges	Primary and secondary diagnoses, primary and secondary procedures	Discharge status, total charges, utilization, readmission (select SID)	No	No
MarketScan	20 Million individuals annually from ~100 private payers	Inpatient and outpatient diagnoses and procedures	Cost, utilization, readmission	Limited	Yes

Abbreviations: MAX, Medicaid Analytic eXtract; VA, Veteran Affairs.

includes more than 100 clinical and nonclinical data elements for each inpatient stay in approximating a 20% stratified sample of community hospitals in the United States. Information includes patient demographics, admission and discharge status, principal and up to 30 secondary diagnosis codes, principal and secondary procedure codes, admission and discharge status, length of stay, and total charges. The SID contains similar data elements but includes 100% inpatient discharge records in participating states. Both NIS and SID contains hospital identifiers that permit linkage with the AHA Annual Survey data and county identifiers for linkage to the Area Resource File. Work is under way to enhance the clinical content of selected state inpatient databases by incorporating electronic laboratory data, hospital-based electronic pharmacy data, electronic prehospital emergency care data, and birth and death certificates.[66]

Commercial claims datasets are also available that contain deidentified, person-specific data on enrollment, clinical utilization, and expenditures across inpatient, outpatient, laboratory, and outpatient pharmacy settings. Thomson Healthcare's MarketScan database, for example, includes data from approximately 100 commercial, Medicare supplemental, and Medicaid payers that can be linked to track detailed patient information across sites, types of providers, and over time.[67] The potential for these databases to be useful for CER is evidenced by a recent study comparing the effectiveness of rosuvastatin with that of other statins for the prevention of cardiovascular events.[68]

Strengths and Limitations of Administrative Data

Administrative data are strengthened by their size and broad population coverage, both of which support analyses in priority populations including racial and ethnic minorities, women, and the elderly. Moreover, administrative include identifiers that enable long-term outcome assessment and the data are relatively efficient to obtain. For heart failure CER, however, administrative data are substantially limited by the absence of clinical data. Few administrative databases include laboratory and pharmacy data, and none include measures of ejection fraction. Although claims-based definitions for systolic dysfunction have high specificity, they have low sensitivity.[69] In addition, administrative data are derived from the process of medical billing, so data elements required for reimbursement and those that generate moderate payments will be reliably coded. Secondary diagnoses and minor procedures are often undercoded, making risk-adjustment difficult.[70] Consequently, a secondary data analysis using administrative data seldom gives a complete clinical picture.

ELECTRONIC HEALTH RECORDS

Electronic health records (EHRs) are longitudinal records of information generated during health care encounters. Typically, EHRs include demographics, progress notes, problems, medications, vital signs, past medical history, and laboratory and radiology results. The use of EHRs for CER holds promise, but many challenges must be addressed. Problem lists and progress notes may be incomplete and provide conflicting information about the patient's clinical status. Reconciling these conflicts is difficult and often requires manual record review. Clinical notes may provide rich detail about signs, symptoms, and treatment decisions, but they are often stored in an unstructured, idiosyncratic form. Information can be extracted manually, but the process is time-consuming and impractical for large studies. Natural language processing shows promise for extracting information in an automated fashion,[71] but much work remains. Finally, information in EHRs is often fragmented, reflecting only the encounters that occurred within the system covered by a given EHR. Except for patients who receive their care within an integrated health care delivery system, absence of information is indistinguishable from absence of disease.

Go and colleagues used administrative and clinical EHR data from Kaiser Permanente of Northern California to assess the comparative effectiveness of different β-blockers among 11,326 adult patients with heart failure. Documentation of ejection fraction was available at 1 site, so a subgroup analysis was performed in patients with left ventricular systolic dysfunction. After adjustment for confounders, the hazard of death was higher for metoprolol tartrate and no β-blocker therapy compared with atenolol but did not differ significantly for patients who received carvedilol.[72] Among 2929 patients with documented left ventricular systolic dysfunction, no significant adjusted differences were observed among the β-blocker uses. Adjusted hazards of rehospitalization for heart failure within 12 months did not differ significantly among treatment groups.[73]

DATABASE LINKAGE

The major challenge in linking different data sources is the availability of identifying information in each dataset. Most heart failure registries do not include direct identifiers such as patient name or Social Security number, although they do include indirect identifiers such as encrypted identifiers and dates of service. Using these indirect identifiers, Hammill and colleagues[74] described a method of linking inpatient clinical registry data to Medicare claims data. The results demonstrated that a combination of indirect identifiers including site, admission date, discharge date, patient age or date of birth, and patient sex could be used to create a robust, linked database. This approach has been used to link the OPTIMIZE-HF, GWTG-HF, ADHERE, and STS registries to longitudinal claims data.

Linking clinical registries and administrative data overcomes the lack of clinical details in administrative database and the absence of long-term assessment in registry data. Importantly, a linked dataset extends the usefulness of both sources of data by providing a more complete picture of the linked patients and the care they receive. Unless the registry and administrative database overlap completely, linkage will limit the analysis population and potentially raise concerns about the generalizability of the study findings. Moreover, reliance on indirect identifiers may result in inaccurate links between databases. External validation is recommended given data availability.[75]

SUMMARY

Existing data sources for heart failure research offer advantages and disadvantages for CER. Clinical registries collect detailed information about disease presentation, treatment, and outcomes on a large number of patients and provide the "real-world" population that is the hallmark of CER. Data are not collected longitudinally, however, and follow-up is often limited. Large administrative datasets provide the broadest population coverage with longitudinal outcomes follow-up but lack clinical detail. Linking clinical registries with other databases to assess longitudinal outcomes holds great promise.

The Federal Coordinating Council for Comparative Effectiveness Research recommends further efforts on longitudinal linking of administrative or EHR-based databases, patient registries, private sector databases (particularly those with commercially insured populations that are not covered under federal and state databases), and other relevant data sources containing pharmacy, laboratory, adverse events, and mortality information. Advancing the infrastructure to provide robust, scientific data resources for patient-centered CER must remain a priority.

REFERENCES

1. Writing Group Members, Lloyd-Jones D, Adams RJ, Brown TM, et al. Heart disease and stroke statistics–2010 update: a report from the American Heart Association. Circulation 2010;121(7):e46–215.
2. West R, Liang L, Fonarow GC, et al. Characterization of heart failure patients with preserved ejection fraction: a comparison between ADHERE-US registry and ADHERE-International registry. Eur J Heart Fail 2011;13(9):945–52.
3. Kociol RD, Hammill BG, Fonarow GC, et al. Generalizability and longitudinal outcomes of a national heart failure clinical registry: comparison of Acute Decompensated Heart Failure National Registry (ADHERE) and non-ADHERE Medicare beneficiaries. Am Heart J 2010;160(5):885–92.
4. Fonarow GC, Abraham WT, Albert NM, et al. Organized program to initiate lifesaving treatment in hospitalized patients with heart failure (OPTIMIZE-HF): rationale and design. Am Heart J 2004;148(1):43–51.
5. Kociol RD, Horton JR, Fonarow GC, et al. Admission, discharge, or change in B-type natriuretic peptide and long-term outcomes: data from Organized Program to Initiate Lifesaving Treatment in Hospitalized Patients with Heart Failure (OPTIMIZE-HF) linked to Medicare claims. Circ Heart Fail 2011; 4(5):628–36.
6. Curtis LH, Greiner MA, Hammill BG, et al. Representativeness of a national heart failure quality-of-care registry: comparison of OPTIMIZE-HF and non-OPTIMIZE-HF Medicare patients. Circ Cardiovasc Qual Outcomes 2009;2(4):377–84.
7. Albert NM, Fonarow GC, Abraham WT, et al. Depression and clinical outcomes in heart failure: an OPTIMIZE-HF analysis. Am J Med 2009;122(4): 366–73.
8. Abraham WT, Fonarow GC, Albert NM, et al. Predictors of in-hospital mortality in patients hospitalized for heart failure: insights from the Organized Program to Initiate Lifesaving Treatment in Hospitalized Patients with Heart Failure (OPTIMIZE-HF). J Am Coll Cardiol 2008;52(5):347–56.
9. Fonarow GC, Abraham WT, Albert NM, et al. Factors identified as precipitating hospital admissions for heart failure and clinical outcomes: findings from OPTIMIZE-HF. Arch Intern Med 2008;168(8):847–54.
10. Fonarow GC, Stough WG, Abraham WT, et al. Characteristics, treatments, and outcomes of patients with preserved systolic function hospitalized for heart failure: a report from the OPTIMIZE-HF Registry. J Am Coll Cardiol 2007;50(8):768–77.
11. Gheorghiade M, Abraham WT, Albert NM, et al. Systolic blood pressure at admission, clinical characteristics, and outcomes in patients hospitalized with acute heart failure. JAMA 2006;296(18):2217–26.
12. Fonarow GC, Abraham WT, Albert NM, et al. Age- and gender-related differences in quality of care and outcomes of patients hospitalized with heart failure (from OPTIMIZE-HF). Am J Cardiol 2009; 104(1):107–15.

13. Fonarow GC, Abraham WT, Albert NM, et al. Dosing of beta-blocker therapy before, during, and after hospitalization for heart failure (from Organized Program to Initiate Lifesaving Treatment in Hospitalized Patients with Heart Failure). Am J Cardiol 2008; 102(11):1524–9.

14. Yancy CW, Abraham WT, Albert NM, et al. Quality of care of and outcomes for African Americans hospitalized with heart failure: findings from the OPTIMIZE-HF (Organized Program to Initiate Lifesaving Treatment in Hospitalized Patients With Heart Failure) registry. J Am Coll Cardiol 2008;51(17):1675–84.

15. Levy PD, Nandyal D, Welch RD, et al. Does aspirin use adversely influence intermediate-term postdischarge outcomes for hospitalized patients who are treated with angiotensin-converting enzyme inhibitors or angiotensin receptor blockers? Findings from Organized Program to Facilitate Life-Saving Treatment in Hospitalized Patients with Heart Failure (OPTIMIZE-HF). Am Heart J 2010;159(2):222–30. e222.

16. Hernandez AF, Hammill BG, Peterson ED, et al. Relationships between emerging measures of heart failure processes of care and clinical outcomes. Am Heart J 2010;159(3):406–13.

17. Hernandez AF, Hammill BG, O'Connor CM, et al. Clinical effectiveness of beta-blockers in heart failure: findings from the OPTIMIZE-HF (Organized Program to Initiate Lifesaving Treatment in Hospitalized Patients with Heart Failure) Registry. J Am Coll Cardiol 2009;53(2):184–92.

18. Fonarow GC, Abraham WT, Albert NM, et al. Influence of beta-blocker continuation or withdrawal on outcomes in patients hospitalized with heart failure: findings from the OPTIMIZE-HF program. J Am Coll Cardiol 2008;52(3):190–9.

19. Fonarow GC, Abraham WT, Albert NM, et al. Association between performance measures and clinical outcomes for patients hospitalized with heart failure. JAMA 2007;297(1):61–70.

20. Hong Y, LaBresh KA. Overview of the American Heart Association "Get with the Guidelines" programs: coronary heart disease, stroke, and heart failure. Crit Pathw Cardiol 2006;5(4):179–86.

21. Kociol RD, Greiner MA, Fonarow GC, et al. Associations of patient demographic characteristics and regional physician density with early physician follow-up among Medicare beneficiaries hospitalized with heart failure. Am J Cardiol 2011;108(7): 985–91.

22. Piccini JP, Hernandez AF, Dai D, et al. Use of cardiac resynchronization therapy in patients hospitalized with heart failure. Circulation 2008;118(9): 926–33.

23. Patel UD, Hernandez AF, Liang L, et al. Quality of care and outcomes among patients with heart failure and chronic kidney disease: a Get With The Guidelines–Heart Failure program study. Am Heart J 2008;156(4):674–81.

24. Horwich TB, Hernandez AF, Liang L, et al. Weekend hospital admission and discharge for heart failure: association with quality of care and clinical outcomes. Am Heart J 2009;158(3):451–8.

25. Piccini JP, Hernandez AF, Zhao X, et al. Quality of care for atrial fibrillation among patients hospitalized for heart failure. J Am Coll Cardiol 2009;54(14):1280–9.

26. Hernandez AF, Fonarow GC, Hammill BG, et al. Clinical effectiveness of implantable cardioverter-defibrillators among Medicare beneficiaries with heart failure. Circ Heart Fail 2010;3(1):7–13.

27. Krantz MJ, Ambardekar AV, Kaltenbach L, et al. Patterns and predictors of evidence-based medication continuation among hospitalized heart failure patients (from Get With the Guidelines-Heart Failure). Am J Cardiol 2011;107(12):1818–23.

28. Gharacholou SM, Hellkamp AS, Hernandez AF, et al. Use and predictors of heart failure disease management referral in patients hospitalized with heart failure: insights from the Get With the Guidelines Program. J Card Fail 2011;17(5):431–9.

29. Hernandez AF, Fonarow GC, Liang L, et al. Sex and racial differences in the use of implantable cardioverter-defibrillators among patients hospitalized with heart failure. JAMA 2007;298(13):1525–32.

30. Klein L, Grau-Sepulveda MV, Bonow RO, et al. Quality of care and outcomes in women hospitalized for heart failure. Circ Heart Fail 2011;4(5):589–98.

31. Thomas KL, Hernandez AF, Dai D, et al. Association of race/ethnicity with clinical risk factors, quality of care, and acute outcomes in patients hospitalized with heart failure. Am Heart J 2011;161(4):746–54.

32. Hernandez AF, Greiner MA, Fonarow GC, et al. Relationship between early physician follow-up and 30-day readmission among Medicare beneficiaries hospitalized for heart failure. JAMA 2010;303(17): 1716–22.

33. Diercks DB, Fonarow GC, Kirk JD, et al. Illicit stimulant use in a United States heart failure population presenting to the emergency department (from the Acute Decompensated Heart Failure National Registry Emergency Module). Am J Cardiol 2008; 102(9):1216–9.

34. Maisel AS, Peacock WF, McMullin N, et al. Timing of immunoreactive B-type natriuretic peptide levels and treatment delay in acute decompensated heart failure: an ADHERE (Acute Decompensated Heart Failure National Registry) analysis. J Am Coll Cardiol 2008;52(7):534–40.

35. Fonarow GC, Heywood JT, Heidenreich PA, et al. Temporal trends in clinical characteristics, treatments, and outcomes for heart failure hospitalizations, 2002 to 2004: findings from Acute Decompensated Heart Failure National Registry (ADHERE). Am Heart J 2007;153(6):1021–8.

36. Yancy CW, Lopatin M, Stevenson LW, et al. Clinical presentation, management, and in-hospital outcomes of patients admitted with acute decompensated heart failure with preserved systolic function: a report from the Acute Decompensated Heart Failure National Registry (ADHERE) Database. J Am Coll Cardiol 2006;47(1):76–84.

37. Fonarow GC, Peacock WF, Phillips CO, et al. Admission B-type natriuretic peptide levels and in-hospital mortality in acute decompensated heart failure. J Am Coll Cardiol 2007;49(19):1943–50.

38. Peacock WF, De Marco T, Fonarow GC, et al. Cardiac troponin and outcome in acute heart failure. N Engl J Med 2008;358(20):2117–26.

39. Fonarow GC, Peacock WF, Horwich TB, et al. Usefulness of B-type natriuretic peptide and cardiac troponin levels to predict in-hospital mortality from ADHERE. Am J Cardiol 2008;101(2):231–7.

40. Heywood JT, Fonarow GC, Costanzo MR, et al. High prevalence of renal dysfunction and its impact on outcome in 118,465 patients hospitalized with acute decompensated heart failure: a report from the ADHERE database. J Card Fail 2007;13(6):422–30.

41. Peacock WF, Fonarow GC, Emerman CL, et al. Impact of early initiation of intravenous therapy for acute decompensated heart failure on outcomes in ADHERE. Cardiology 2007;107(1):44–51.

42. Peacock WF, Hollander JE, Diercks DB, et al. Morphine and outcomes in acute decompensated heart failure: an ADHERE analysis. Emerg Med J 2008;25(4):205–9.

43. Abraham WT, Adams KF, Fonarow GC, et al. In-hospital mortality in patients with acute decompensated heart failure requiring intravenous vasoactive medications: an analysis from the Acute Decompensated Heart Failure National Registry (ADHERE). J Am Coll Cardiol 2005;46(1):57–64.

44. National Cardiovascular Data Registry. Available at: http://www.ncdr.com/WebNCDR/NCDRDocuments/FAQ%20ICD.pdf. Accessed December 12, 2010.

45. Hammill SC, Kremers MS, Kadish AH, et al. Review of the ICD registry's third year, expansion to include lead data and pediatric ICD procedures, and role for measuring performance. Heart Rhythm 2009;6(9):1397–401.

46. Hammill SC, Kremers MS, Stevenson LW, et al. Review of the registry's fourth year, incorporating lead data and pediatric ICD procedures, and use as a national performance measure. Heart Rhythm 2010;7(9):1340–5.

47. Peterson ED, Roe MT, Rumsfeld JS, et al. A call to ACTION (acute coronary treatment and intervention outcomes network). Circ Cardiovasc Qual Outcomes 2009;2(5):491–9.

48. Peterson ED, Roe MT, Chen AY, et al. The NCDR ACTION Registry–GWTG: transforming contemporary acute myocardial infarction clinical care. Heart 2010;96(22):1798–802.

49. Clark RE. The STS National Database: alive, well, and growing. Ann Thorac Surg 1991;52(1):5.

50. Jacobs JP, Haan CK, Edwards FH, et al. The rationale for incorporation of HIPAA compliant unique patient, surgeon, and hospital identifier fields in the STS database. Ann Thorac Surg 2008;86(3):695–8.

51. O'Brien SM, Shahian DM, Filardo G, et al. The Society of Thoracic Surgeons 2008 cardiac surgery risk models: part 2–isolated valve surgery. Ann Thorac Surg 2009;88(Suppl 1):S23–42.

52. Shahian DM, O'Brien SM, Filardo G, et al. The Society of Thoracic Surgeons 2008 cardiac surgery risk models: part 1–coronary artery bypass grafting surgery. Ann Thorac Surg 2009;88(Suppl 1):S2–22.

53. Shahian DM, O'Brien SM, Filardo G, et al. The Society of Thoracic Surgeons 2008 cardiac surgery risk models: part 3–valve plus coronary artery bypass grafting surgery. Ann Thorac Surg 2009;88(Suppl 1):S43–62.

54. Dhruva SS, Redberg RF. Variations between clinical trial participants and Medicare beneficiaries in evidence used for Medicare national coverage decisions. Arch Intern Med 2008;168(2):136–40.

55. Berger JS, Melloni C, Wang TY, et al. Reporting and representation of race/ethnicity in published randomized trials. Am Heart J 2009;158(5):742–7.

56. Medicare Enrollment Reports 2006. Centers for Medicare & Medicaid Services. Available at: https://www.cms.gov/MedicareEnRpts/. Accessed March 19, 2011.

57. 2009 Annual Report of the Boards of Trustees of the Federal Hospital Insurance and Federal Supplementary Medical Insurance Trust Funds. Available at: http://www.cms.gov/Research-Statistics-Data-and-Systems/Statistics-Trends-and-Reports/ReportsTrustFunds/downloads/tr2009.pdf. Accessed October 11, 2012.

58. Centers for Medicare & Medicaid Services. Medicare provider analysis and review (MEDPAR) file. Available at: http://www4.cms.gov/IdentifiableDataFiles/05_MedicareProviderAnalysisandReviewFile.asp. Accessed March 21, 2011.

59. Centers for Medicare & Medicaid Services. Medicaid & CHIP program information eligibility. Available at: http://www.medicaid.gov/Medicaid-CHIP-Program-Information/By-Topics/Eligibility/Eligibility.html. Accessed April 30, 2012.

60. Centers for Medicare & Medicaid Services. Medicaid Analytic eXtract (MAX) general information. Available at: http://www.medicaid.gov/Medicaid-CHIP-Program-Information/By-Topics/Data-and-Systems/MAX/MAX-General-Information.html. Accessed March 21, 2011.

61. Kramer JM, Curtis LH, Dupree CS, et al. Comparative effectiveness of beta-blockers in elderly patients with heart failure. Arch Intern Med 2008;168(22):2422–8 [discussion: 2428–32].

62. National Center for Veterans Analysis and Statistics. Utilization: Selected Veterans Health Administration Characteristics: FY2002 to FY2011. Available at: http://www.va.gov/vetdata/Utilization.asp. Accessed October 17, 2012.

63. United States Department of Veterans Affairs. VA Information Resource Center. VA Data Sources. Available at: http://www.virec.research.va.gov/DataSourcesName/DataNames.htm. Accessed March 21, 2011.

64. Desai RJ, Ashton CM, Deswal A, et al. Comparative effectiveness of individual angiotensin receptor blockers on risk of mortality in patients with chronic heart failure. Pharmacoepidemiol Drug Saf 2012; 21(3):233–40.

65. HCUP Databases. Healthcare Cost and Utilization Project (HCUP). Rockville (MD): Agency for Healthcare Research and Quality; 2010. Available at: www.hcup-us.ahrq.gov/databases.jsp. Accessed October 11, 2012.

66. Data Innovations. Healthcare Cost and Utilization Project (HCUP). 2010. Available at: www.hcup-us.ahrq.gov/datainnovations/grants.jsp. Accessed April 30, 2012.

67. 2011 Thomson Reuters. MarketScan Research Databases. Available at: http://thomsonreuters.com/products_services/healthcare/healthcare_products/pharmaceuticals/mktscan_res_db/. Accessed March 21, 2011.

68. Motsko SP, Russmann S, Ming EE, et al. Effectiveness of rosuvastatin compared to other statins for the prevention of cardiovascular events-a cohort study in 395 039 patients from clinical practice. Pharmacoepidemiol Drug Saf 2009; 18(12):1214–22.

69. Li Q, Glynn RJ, Dreyer NA, et al. Validity of claims-based definitions of left ventricular systolic dysfunction in Medicare patients. Pharmacoepidemiol Drug Saf 2011;20(7):700–8.

70. Quan H, Parsons GA, Ghali WA. Validity of information on comorbidity derived rom ICD-9-CCM administrative data. Med Care 2002;40(8):675–85.

71. Murff HJ, FitzHenry F, Matheny ME, et al. Automated identification of postoperative complications within an electronic medical record using natural language processing. JAMA 2011;306(8):848–55.

72. Go AS, Yang J, Gurwitz JH, et al. Comparative effectiveness of different beta-adrenergic antagonists on mortality among adults with heart failure in clinical practice. Arch Intern Med 2008;168(22):2415–21.

73. Go AS, Yang J, Gurwitz JH, et al. Comparative effectiveness of beta-adrenergic antagonists (atenolol, metoprolol tartrate, carvedilol) on the risk of rehospitalization in adults with heart failure. Am J Cardiol 2007;100(4):690–6.

74. Hammill BG, Hernandez AF, Peterson ED, et al. Linking inpatient clinical registry data to Medicare claims data using indirect identifiers. Am Heart J 2009; 157(6):995–1000.

75. Méray N, Reitsma JB, Ravelli AC, et al. Probabilistic record linkage is a valid and transparent tool to combine databases without a patient identification number. J Clin Epidemiol 2007;60(9):883–91.

End Points for Comparative Effectiveness Research in Heart Failure

Larry A. Allen, MD, MHS[a],*, John A. Spertus, MD, MPH[b]

KEYWORDS

- End points • Congestive heart failure • Comparative effectiveness research • Study design

KEY POINTS

- With the increasing availability of therapeutic strategies and the growing complexity of health care delivery, objective evidence of the tangible benefits of different approaches to care is needed, especially for patients with heart failure, a resource-intensive disease.
- Few well-proven therapies exist for patients with acute decompensation or for patients with normal left ventricular ejection fraction.
- Comparative effectiveness research (CER) offers an important avenue for making progress in the field; however, CER, like any well-designed research program, requires articulation of clinically important outcomes to be compared.
- For patients with heart failure, end-point measures that capture the totality of potential benefits and risks for alternative therapeutic approaches must be developed.
- For one therapeutic approach to be considered superior to another, it must make patients live longer, make them feel better, or save money without adversely affecting the other 2 goals.
- Importantly, these outcomes must be measured directly and surrogates should be avoided, even if such surrogates seem to be associated with clinically meaningful, patient-centered outcomes.

INTRODUCTION

As medical therapies continue to expand and the delivery of health care becomes increasingly complex, there is a growing need to inform patients, clinicians, and policy makers of the relative value of alternative treatment options. Comparative effectiveness research (CER) is emerging as a central approach to help guide health care decisions by providing data about the relative safety and effectiveness of various therapeutic approaches. Although CER offers the hope of improving the quality of our health care delivery system, it is a science in rapid evolution.

The process of comparing one therapy with another involves comparing how various approaches differentially affect clinically meaningful outcomes. From the patient, clinician, and societal perspectives, the value of a therapy stems from its impact on 3 main concepts: does the therapy make patients live longer? Does the therapy make patients feel better? Or does the therapy save resources? Although survival, quality of life, and cost may seem on face value to be straightforward concepts, accurate assessment and interpretation of these end points is complex. Researchers must choose which measures to

Disclosures: Dr John Spertus owns the copyright to the Kansas City Cardiomyopathy Questionnaire. There are no other relevant conflicts to report.
[a] Division of Cardiology, University of Colorado School of Medicine, Anschutz Medical Center, Academic Office 1, 12631 East 17th Avenue, Mailstop B130, Aurora, CO 80045, USA; [b] Saint Luke's Mid America Heart Institute, University of Missouri, 4401 Wornall Road, Kansas City, MO 64111, USA
* Corresponding author.
E-mail address: larry.allen@ucdenver.edu

Heart Failure Clin 9 (2013) 15–28
http://dx.doi.org/10.1016/j.hfc.2012.09.002

collect, how to collect those measures efficiently and accurately, and how to weigh competing measures against one another.

Heart failure exemplifies the issues around end points in CER.[1–3] The heart failure syndrome includes patients with diverse presentations and pathophysiology, usually in combination with high degrees of comorbidity and advanced age. Heart failure is the leading cause of hospitalization and rehospitalization among older adults in the United States, at a direct cost of more than $40 billion per year.[4] Heart failure remains a common, morbid, and resource-intensive disease, in part because few treatment approaches have been shown to be efficacious for patients with acute decompensation[5] or for patients with heart failure and normal left ventricular ejection fraction (LVEF).[6] In addition, because heart failure is a highly symptomatic disease, and because many attempted therapies have failed to improve mortality, there is increasing interest in assessing effectiveness for a wide range of end points that reflect quality of life and cost. Heart failure research is marked by significant heterogeneity in end-point assessment.

CER for patients with heart failure needs to develop end points that encompass the totality of potential benefits (and risks) for alternative therapeutic approaches, including relieving symptoms, improving overall quality of life, limiting hospitalization (a surrogate for costs), and prolonging survival. Greater standardization of end points across CER studies would allow therapies to be more easily compared and prioritized by patients, clinicians, and payers. In this review, the potential CER end-point domains from both a clinical and a research perspective are discussed, the wide variety of end points used in completed and ongoing CER studies are summarized, and steps are suggested for greater standardization of end points across CER for patients with heart failure.

DEFINITIONS AND OVERALL CONSIDERATIONS

End points in medical research are specific, identifiable, downstream events or changes in a patient's condition. Clinically meaningful end points should be evident to and important to patients (eg, not laboratory measures). In addition, ideal end points should be unambiguous, consistent, easy to obtain, inexpensive to measure, sensitive to the processes of care that they are designed to reflect, and simple to understand. Heart failure is typically progressive, systemic in its effects, highly symptomatic, and lethal. Therefore, a wide range of end-point options are available (**Table 1**). When considering end-point design for

heart failure studies, a general framework of the disease process should be taken into account.

Although there are diverse and complex pathophysiologic disturbances in heart failure, including left ventricular remodeling and neurohormonal dysregulation, the outcomes of mortality and health status (symptoms, function, and quality of life) are relatively constant across the spectrum of the heart failure syndrome. The definition of heart failure as a syndrome, rather than a disease, underscores the concept that multiple pathophysiologic disturbances lead to similar health status limitations and mortality. Regardless of its cause, patients with heart failure follow a similar, albeit variable, clinical course. **Fig. 1** outlines a schematic approach to the syndrome. Patients are often diagnosed with heart failure after suffering with undiagnosed symptoms for some time (stage 1). After initial diagnosis and treatment, they often enter a period of relative stability (stage 2), punctuated with periodic but increasing episodes of decompensation (stage 3), resulting in acute care/hospitalizations. At some point, they enter a terminal trajectory (stage 4), at which stage, heart transplantation of left ventricular assist devices can be considered for a select group of patients with reduced LVEF to move them to a previous phase of their trajectory (eg, stage 2). However, a terminal stage emerges (stage 5), for which the therapeutic goals shift toward comfort care in preparation for death. This progressive course may be truncated at any point by sudden cardiac death, which is common among patients with heart failure and reduced LVEF. This schematic, originally created by Dale Renlund and colleagues, highlights the variable, but generally progressive course of the disease.[7] It also highlights clinically important outcomes (health status, hospitalizations, transplant or device therapy, and death) that can be measured throughout the disease course.

VITAL STATUS

Vital status (variably expressed as mortality or survival) is of unquestioned importance as a clinically relevant end point. Patients with symptomatic heart failure have an average survival of less than 5 years,[8] so vital status measures are particularly important in assessing treatments for these patients. Unlike many other end points, all-cause mortality is objective, easy to assess, and can often be obtained retrospectively. Consequently, mortality is generally considered the gold standard of clinical end points, and it is the most commonly reported end point in CER studies.

Vital status can be obtained through a variety of mechanisms, including queries to families, to

Table 1
Categories of potential end points for CER in heart failure

Category	Specific End Points	Advantages	Disadvantages

Vital status (quantity of life)	Mortality
	  All-cause
	  Cardiovascular
	  Pump failure
	  Sudden death
		The gold standard: highly objective, easy to obtain accurately on patients over long-term follow-up	Number likely needs to be large and follow-up long; therapies that improve many patients, especially with advanced heart failure, may value trade quantity for quality of life

Health status (quality of life)	Health status questionnaires
	  Disease-specific
	  Generic
	Utilities
	NYHA functional classification
	Symptom scales
		By definition reflects how patients feel, making them clinically relevant	Must be obtained directly from patient, prospectively; time-consuming questionnaires

Cost (resource use)	Inflation-adjusted dollars
	  Direct vs indirect
	  Fixed vs variable
		An objective outcome with patient and societal importance; the numerator in cost-effectiveness analyses used to determining the relative value of care, which is a major goal of CER	Must interpret in context of therapy effectiveness (cost-effectiveness/cost-utility measures are more meaningful than cost alone); it is difficult to directly capture all costs; often requires multiple assumptions that are not well characterized; critically dependent on the perspective taken (ie, patient, payer, society)

Mixed (hospitalization)	Index admission Length of stay Readmissions Total days in hospital	Important clinical measure of cost but also closely linked to health status and predictor or mortality; easy to measure; relatively objective	Variable between providers, institutions, and countries as standards for admission and dischargability do not exist; surrogate for health status
Surrogates	Vital signs Blood tests Imaging studies	Typically objective; short follow-up needed; continuous variables; allow for smaller, shorter, early-phase studies	Frequently surrogate measures do not relate to clinically relevant events
Composites	Combined Ranked	May increase power; may help capture a wider range of important outcome domains; accounts for competing events (ie, death) rather than censoring such events	More difficult to interpret; least important component often drives result
Safety	Medication side effects Procedural complications	May be less susceptible to treatment selection biases and confounding	May require noninferiority statistical approaches to say that one approach is no more dangerous than another; some side effects are rare and occur far out from start of intervention, requiring alternatives to RCT for detection (phase IV surveillance)

Abbreviations: NYHA, New York Heart Association; RCT, randomized controlled trial.

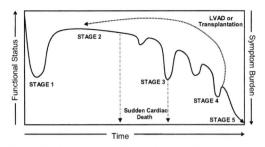

Fig. 1. Clinical course of heart failure, showing some of the events that may be captured as end points. (*Adapted from* Goodlin SJ, Hauptman PJ, Arnold R, et al. Consensus statement: palliative and supportive care in advanced heart failure. J Card Fail 2004; 10(3):204; with permission.)

health plans, or to administrative records (State death certificates, the National Death Index, and Social Security Death Master File), if adequate patient identifiers (eg, social security numbers) are available.

However, controversy remains about whether it is preferable to measure all-cause or disease-specific mortality.[9] All-cause mortality has the advantage of being completely objective and has a higher overall event rate than disease-specific mortality. However, the critique of all-cause mortality is that it includes events that are unlikely to be responsive to the heart failure treatments in question, so the signal of treatment efficacy may be obscured by the noise of other causes for death. Therefore, disease-specific event rates related to the specific mechanism of action of the therapy (eg, sudden death in defibrillator studies) are more likely to have a treatment effect, assuming that the mechanism of action of the therapy is understood. Mode of death may also significantly influence quality of life and cost in the last months of life (eg, sudden cardiac death compared with progressive pump failure). Therapies that reduce one mode of death may inadvertently increase another (eg, arrhythmic death vs nonarrhythmic death with the implantation of defibrillators immediately after myocardial infarction),[10] and thus even if a disease-specific cause of death is chosen, all-cause mortality should still be reported. Data from heart failure trials among patients with reduced LVEF have found that most postdischarge deaths are cardiovascular in nature,[11,12] even among older patients and those with normal LVEF.[13,14] If disease-specific mortality is believed to be an important end point, adjudication of cause-specific mortality is needed.[15] Death certificates are notoriously inaccurate.[16] Therefore, determining deaths from cardiovascular causes, heart failure, progressive pump failure, sudden

cardiac death, and so forth invariably requires some active interpretation of the clinical events leading up to death. This interpretation necessitates prospective standardized capture of physician-determined cause of death or detailed chart reviews to adjudicate cause of death. When patients die outside the hospital, arbitrary rules must be established to assign the cause of their demise; often clearly noncardiovascular causes of death are labeled as such (eg, trauma or metastatic cancer) and then all other deaths are presumed to be cardiovascular in nature. All of these factors should be considered when deciding whether or not to measure disease-specific mortality. In the end, observational CER studies, especially those using administrative data, lack detailed clinical information, so all-cause mortality is the preferred end point.

Despite its obvious importance, death as a single end point has the disadvantage of limited statistical power and misses other dimensions of outcome important to patients. Although heart failure is a highly lethal condition, use of mortality as the end point still requires large sample sizes, longer follow-up, and large treatment effect to show significant differences. The heterogeneity of the population, the high prevalence of contributing comorbidities, and the failure of many therapies to improve survival have discouraged the use of mortality as the lone end point in clinical trials. Although some administrative heart failure databases, which include tens of thousands of patients, can overcome issues of statistical power that plague clinical trials, they cannot address many of the other methodological concerns (eg, treatment selection bias, confounding) present in observational studies of treatment effect.

HEALTH STATUS

A major limitation in the current focus on survival is that it incorrectly presumes that all survival represents an equally favorable outcome. Health status (symptoms, function, and quality of life) are primary concerns for patients. Multiple studies have shown that nearly half of patients with heart failure would make health care decisions that improve their quality of life even if it reduced their life expectancy.[17–19] Near the end of life, health status may be given even greater priority. Although traditionally considered a soft outcome, because it comes from patients, rather than an objective test, the reproducibility and sensitivity to clinical change of standardized questionnaires are better than many other modalities of quantifying patients' function.[20] Yet, despite the availability of validated measures, a principal challenge in conducting

CER with health status as an outcome has been the lack of systematic quantification of health status in clinical studies, observational research, and clinical care.

Survival and quality of life both represent critical patient-centered outcomes, but their practical use as end points in research is disparate. Whereas all-cause mortality is a simple dichotomous measure that can usually be obtained retrospectively, quality-of-life measures must be prospectively obtained via direct input from the patient. Thus, although quality of life is clearly an important end point, its use in CER studies has been limited because of these logistical limitations. Because health care value is receiving increasing attention and because value cannot be determined without including some measure of quality of life (eg, resource use per quality-adjusted life years [cost/QALY] for cost-utility analyses), CER studies are likely to increasingly involve assessments of quality of life.

Methods for Assessing Health Status

Heart failure affects patients' lives in several ways. Although many use the term quality of life to encompass all outcomes beyond survival, we consider it to be a distinct domain and prefer the term health status to refer to the combination of domains in which a disease can affect patients. These domains include the following: the symptoms of disease; the physical, emotional, and social limitations associated with these symptoms and patients' quality of life; and the discrepancy between patients' current symptoms and functioning and how they expect to be feeling and functioning. **Fig. 2** outlines a framework for understanding how heart failure can affect the health status of afflicted patients.

In clinical research studies, there are several methods for quantifying the impact of the disease on patients' health status. Prototypical examples of health status measures are provided in **Table 2**. An important consideration is whether generic health status measures, which quantify a patients' overall health, or disease-specific measures, which focus on the clinical syndrome of heart failure, should be used.

Disease-Specific Health Status Measures

Although there are a myriad of potential causes for heart failure, patients are unaware of these pathophysiologic mechanisms. What they are aware of are the symptoms of fatigue, shortness of breath, and edema. These symptoms, in turn, can limit their physical and social activities and impair their emotional functioning. As noted earlier, the degree to which their symptoms and functional limitations differ from their expectations for their health, the worse their quality of life is.

The most common metric of the impact of heart failure on patients is the New York Heart Association (NYHA) functional classification.[21] This 4-class measure is the most commonly used measure of patients' symptoms and function in clinical practice and in research, but suffers from several critical limitations. First, it reflects patients' health status from physicians' perspectives and not patients themselves. Second, its validity and reproducibility have been questioned.[22,23] Less commonly used metrics, particularly in trials of acute heart failure, are single-item measures of dyspnea or global health.[24] There are no validated instruments for dyspnea assessment that are accurate, reliable, reproducible between observers, and sensitive to acute changes in dyspnea.[25] Instead, an assortment of poorly validated instruments are used assessing dyspnea, including Likert scales, visual analogue scales, and more complicated measures.[26,27] Patterns of dyspnea resolution are significantly affected by choice of response instrument.[28]

Several disease-specific health status measures have been developed for patients with heart failure,

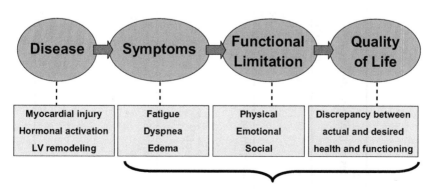

The Range of Health Status

Fig. 2. A conceptual model of health status.

Table 2
Examples of health-related quality-of-life instruments that may be used in CER

	Description	Scoring	Advantages	Disadvantages
Utilities	Quantification of strength of preference for current health status vs perfect health status with risk of early death		Can be readily combined with survival; necessary for cost-effectiveness analyses	Difficult to obtain from patients
Standard gamble[42]		Percent risk of immediate death a patient is willing to accept for return to perfect health	Standard method for determination of utilities	
Time trade-off[43]		Percent of remaining life span a person is willing to trade away for perfect health	More easily interpreted by clinicians and patients	
Generic Health Status Measures	Assessments of patients' symptoms, functioning, and quality of life		Easily compared across studies; map to utilities	Insensitive to important clinical changes in patients with heart failure
EQ-5D[37]	5 dimensions Mobility Self-care Usual activities Pain/discomfort Anxiety/depression	Each item: no, some, extreme; score −1 to 1		
HUI[38]	Multiple dimensions depending on version (vision, hearing, speech, ambulation, dexterity, emotion, cognition, pain, cognitive, self-care, fertility)	Score 0–1		

			Sensitive to important clinical changes	Have not been mapped to utilities
SF-36[40]	8 dimensions Physical functioning Role limitations physical Bodily pain General health Vitality Mental health Role limitations emotional Social functioning	Each item: yes or no; score 0–100		
Disease-Specific Health Status Measures	Assessments of patients' symptoms, functioning, and quality of life			
MLwHF[29]	21-items Physical Mental	105–0 (higher scores worse)		
KCCQ[30]	23-items in 6 domains: Physical limitation Symptoms Quality of life Social interference Self-efficacy Overall summary	0–100 (higher scores better)		

Abbreviations: EQ-5D, EuroQol; HUI, Health Utilities Index; KCCQ, Kansas City Cardiomyopathy Questionnaire; MLwHF, Minnesota Living with Heart Failure Questionnaire; SF, short form.

of which the most commonly used are the Minnesota Living with Heart Failure (MLwHF) questionnaire[29] and the Kansas City Cardiomyopathy Questionnaire (KCCQ).[30] The MLwHF provides an overall summary score, with a physical and mental component. The KCCQ follows the framework in **Fig. 2**, with specific scales to quantify symptoms, physical and social function, and quality of life. The KCCQ also has a scale to measure self-efficacy, the degree to which patients are confident in managing their heart failure, and changes in symptoms over the past 2 weeks. The KCCQ has been shown to be more sensitive to changes in clinical status than EuroQol (EQ-5D) and its visual analogue scale, 12-item short form questionnaire (SF-12), 6-minute walk test, and NYHA functional classification.[31] Although the KCCQ was designed to quantify patient-centered outcomes, it has also been associated with prognosis and costs.[32–36] Yet, despite the psychometric and prognostic validity of the MLwHF and KCCQ, they are seldom used in clinical trials, observational registries, or routine clinical care.[20]

Generic Health Status Measures

In parallel to disease-specific measures that explicitly seek to quantify how the heart failure syndrome affects patients' lives, researchers have also developed generic measures of health status. These instruments quantify the overall health of patients, including heart failure and all other comorbidities. Common examples include the EQ-5D,[37] the Health Utilities Index (HUI),[38] the Duke Activity Status Index (DASI),[39] and the SF-12 or 36-item short form questionnaires (SF-36).[40] Although the advantage of these measures is that they can permit comparisons between heart-failure treatments and treatments for other diseases on a common scale, they are less sensitive to important clinical changes than disease-specific measures.[41]

Utilities

To perform cost-effectiveness or decision analyses, in which an explicit goal is to combine survival and the quality of that survival, there is a need to distill patients' health status to a single number (a utility) that can be used to determine QALY of survival. A utility is thus a quantification of the strength of an individual's preference for any of several possible outcomes of a decision.[42] This conceptualization of utility has been used widely in economics and public policy, but medical applications have been more limited. In a medical context, a utility rates health status by measuring the value that an individual places on their current

health state. A utility is best measured through an exercise, such as the standard gamble, in which a patient is asked to choose between accepting their current state of health and undergoing a procedure that results in either immediate death or perfect health. The risk of death associated with the procedure is varied until the patient is indifferent in a choice between current health state and taking a chance on the procedure. These sequential gambles on immediate death versus perfect health yield a risk of dying that can be interpreted as the percentage of perfect health that a patient currently has. For example, if a patient is willing to accept a 15% chance of immediate death to be restored to perfect health, then their current utility is 85% of perfect health. A simpler method, the time trade-off (TTO), was developed as an alternative to the standard gamble specifically for use in medical applications.[43,44] It seems to be more easily interpreted by clinicians and patients, and gives results quantitatively similar to the standard gamble. Although utility measures are grounded in theory, they are difficult to assess reliably, and hence are seldom collected in clinical studies. Smaller samples are generally assessed to support modeling approaches that estimate the cost-effectiveness of alternative therapies.

An alternative approach to directly assessing patients' utilities is to use generic health status measures that have been mapped to utility weights. Examples include the EQ-5D, HUI, DASI, and SF-36. Their scoring is based on a correlation of questionnaire results with standard gamble or TTO results from community-based samples, often those without the disease of interest. Although there has been general acceptance that the utility weights assigned to the EQ-5D are reasonable representations of society's values for various health states, other approaches have gained less acceptance and none of these methods represents patients' perspectives of their disease well.

COST

Intensity of resource use is a highly relevant outcome in CER, which aims to determine the relative value of different care approaches. With growing pressure to control health care expenditures, cost end points are likely to become increasingly collected and reported. However, the cost of care can be assessed only in the context of the outcomes of that care. Furthermore, the total costs of a therapy, including its impact on downstream costs, need to be known to provide a fair picture of the value of various health care options.[45] Therefore, the goal must be to compare the relative value of various health care options, by combining total costs with a comprehensive assessment of benefits and risks within the framework of cost-effectiveness analyses.

Unlike the existing decentralized coverage decision process in the United States, most industrialized countries have been more interested in confronting cost-effectiveness from a national level. The National Institute for Health and Clinical Excellence (NICE), a special authority of the National Health Service in England and Wales, effectively requires cost and utility data to be collected in the drug development process. NICE provides an example of how cost-effectiveness data may be used to compare the relative value of therapies and guide coverage decisions.[46] Although Americans have generally shown less tolerance for such centralized regulation, there is growing interest in the United States to reduce health care utilization though free choice in response to pricing mechanisms.[47] Again, CER that collects cost data as an end point is essential to help guide such decisions.

Studies that collect data on resource use and cost are difficult to perform and complex to interpret. Because cost studies generally try to sum the totality of resource use in order to assess the relative efficiency of alternative health care interventions, they require consideration of a wide range of end points. These end points include both medical and nonmedical costs (eg, loss of work, transportation). In addition, which resources are included in the end point of cost are highly dependent on the perspective chosen. For example, costs realized are different for the patient versus the health system versus the insurance payer versus society, at large. Therefore, before an economic evaluation begins, the perspective of the study must be determined, because it has important implications for end-point selection and collection. In interpreting CER with cost data, costs assigned to various resources that are collected as end points may change rapidly over time. The article on health economics issues in CER elsewhere in this issue by Kazi and Mark, addresses many of these themes in greater detail.

HOSPITALIZATION

Much of the burden of heart failure occurs around acute care for decompensation. There are now more than 1 million heart failure hospitalizations annually in the United States alone,[4] and approximately 70% of total direct costs are attributable to inpatient care.[48] Hospitalization is typically prompted by severe symptoms. Most patients do not wish to be in hospital. Iatrogenic complications are common. Recurrent hospitalization is itself a strong marker of subsequent adverse outcomes. Therefore, hospitalization is an event that captures both cost and health status, and is a strong surrogate for subsequent mortality, but does not fit neatly into a single category of clinically relevant end points.

Hospitalization can be characterized in a variety of ways. Some studies use first hospitalization as a single time to event measure. For patients who have already been hospitalized for heart failure (a common eligibility criteria or point of capture for many CER studies), readmission may be the end point of interest, and these specific rehospitalization events have received particular attention recently. The end point of rehospitalization is paradoxically related to the length of stay of the index hospitalization, because patients with prolonged index hospitalizations have less time at risk for rehospitalization from the time of index admission. More comprehensive measures of hospitalization may include total number of hospitalizations over some period or total days of hospitalization, as are needed in cost analyses. In addition, the issues of cause-specific versus any hospitalization relate to this outcome, as discussed earlier for mortality. Regardless of the specific hospitalization end point chosen, hospitalization should be considered in the context of overall mortality, because patients who do not survive are not at risk for hospitalization.

Hospitalization end points may be substantially affected by social preferences and regional differences in practice patterns. For example, length of stay for heart-failure hospitalization in European counties is approximately twice that in the United States.[49] In addition, the increased use of short-stay holding units in emergency departments and the use of intravenous medications in heart-failure clinics can confound the definition of hospitalization. New federal policies have been designed to reduce readmission rates.

SAFETY

The difference between effectiveness and safety is in some ways a semantic one, because both represent clinical outcomes that are important to patients and are believed to be influenced by the therapeutic option being tested. A single end point (eg, death or hospitalization) may be prevented in some patients yet caused in others through the application of a therapy, such that many end points are both effectiveness and safety measures. (An additional advantage of using all-cause mortality or readmissions is that this end point more clearly captures events that are a consequence of adverse outcomes attributable to the safety of the intervention, as opposed to its efficacy.) However, some end points (eg, allergic reaction to a drug, procedural complication) are more clearly undesired side effects of the therapy that are best thought of from a safety perspective. The nature of safety end points may make them less susceptible to treatment selection biases, and therefore more amenable to observational CER approaches.

Given the history of drug development in heart failure, the overall safety profile of new therapies has become an issue of significant concern. In particular, when the focus of a therapy is short-term symptom relief without a long-term benefit on morbidity or mortality (as has commonly been tested in therapies for acute heart failure), establishing that this does not occur at the expense of longer-term safety is critical. In this sense, safety end points are effectively noninferiority measures, requiring specific statistical approaches in order to establish noninferiority with a prespecified equivalence boundary.[50] Evaluation of safety for new therapies or approaches to care should be guided by an understanding of the therapy's mechanism of the therapy as well as by signals from earlier clinical study. This evaluation requires testing specific safety hypotheses with the appropriate sample size, which reasonably balances the desire to limit the risk for potential postapproval adverse events with the need for efficient pathways for evaluating new therapies.[51] The degree of risk that must be ruled out in order to declare a treatment safe should be related to the degree and type of benefit (ie, a drug that improves short-term symptoms only may be held to a higher standard of safety than one that improves mortality).

SURROGATES

A surrogate end point is defined by the US Food and Drug Administration as "a laboratory measurement or physical sign that is used in therapeutic trials as a substitute for a clinically meaningful end point that is a direct measure of how a patient feels, functions, or survives and is expected to predict the effect of the therapy."[52] In order to be valid, a surrogate end point should meet clearly defined criteria: (1) the surrogate must be in the causal pathway from the intervention to the clinically relevant outcome, as reflected by a strong association between the surrogate and the target; and (2) there must be no important effects of the intervention on the outcome that are not mediated through or captured by the surrogate.[51] Because it is challenging to establish that these criteria are met, regulatory agencies have generally required that new therapies address

clinically relevant outcomes before approval, and major policy decisions that favor one therapy over another should also be based on CER data that relate to clinically meaningful findings.

The history of drug development in heart failure has been marked by recurrent failure of surrogate end points to accurately predict clinical outcomes in larger efficacy trials. Improved hemodynamics and increased diuresis have not correlated with more robust clinical end points.[53] Recent concerns about previous well-accepted surrogate end points (glucose level, cholesterol level, and vascular intimal-medial thickness) have raised the criticism of surrogate end points to a new level.[54–58] Still, surrogate outcomes continue to have an important role in the development and evaluation of health care therapies, because they often provide a more immediate manifestation of effect and typically allow for shorter and smaller studies. Consequently, early-phase clinical studies using surrogate end points are necessary to guide the design of larger studies. Some surrogate end points deserve particular mention in the design of heart-failure CER.

Many surrogates used in heart-failure studies relate to estimates of cardiac function and remodeling. For patients with reduced LVEF, improvements in cardiac imaging parameters, particularly left ventricular volumes, have correlated well with long-term hard outcomes. However, ventricular reconstruction surgery does not seem to improve outcomes, even although it directly improves the surrogate.[59] Hemodynamic parameters and natriuretic peptides share similar properties to cardiac imaging surrogate markers; experience with nesiritide[60,61] and levosimendan[62,63] shows that improvements in B-type natriuretic peptide and pulmonary-capillary wedge pressure do not necessarily correlate with clinically meaningful outcomes.

The interaction between heart failure and the kidney has become a topic of substantially increased interest in recent years.[64] Worsening renal function in patients with heart failure has been shown to be a powerful predictor of adverse outcomes, and progressive renal failure leads to meaningful clinical events, such as worsening fluid retention and initiation of dialysis. Many recent therapies for heart failure have targeted renal preservation as an end point.[65]

Yet all commonly used surrogates, such as serum creatinine, LVEF, or B-type natriuretic peptide level, are only important insofar as they illuminate the mechanisms of disease progression and can highlight new pathways for which additional therapeutic interventions might be designed and tested. It is the clinically important outcomes of survival, quality of life, and cost that should guide therapeutic decisions. Given the pitfalls of relying on surrogate end points, surrogates should be hypothesis generating and confirmed in studies that directly measure differences in outcomes.

COMBINING END POINTS

There is no single end point that accurately captures the totality of the patient experience with heart failure. Thus, substantial interest exists for combining end points in order to measure the impact of interventions on the various domains of possible benefit. One method for addressing these issues is the use of multiple end points in some type of combination.

Composite end points attempt to combine the various aspects of the experience of heart failure into a single integrated measure. Some end points can be naturally combined into a single end point, if there is a common unit of value to allow for comparison. Examples include the combination of resource use into a single cost measure or the melding of survival and quality of life into QALYs. However, most end points are not so easily condensed. More commonly, a composite end point simply combines separate events into one category. A frequently used combined end point is "time to death or first hospitalization." A more nuanced combination is "days alive and out of the hospital."[66] The theoretic advantage of this latter end point is that it combines mortality, length of stay of the index hospitalization, and the burden of subsequent hospitalizations into a single end point. However, such combinations fundamentally suffer from equating different outcomes (ie, death and hospital admission are not equal in the eyes of most patients). Composite end points may be more appropriate when either of 2 end points trigger a similar response. For example, many decisions about advanced heart-failure therapies are driven by either high risk for death or persistently unfavorable quality of life rather than only one or the other. Therefore, patients at high risk for either end point may warrant consideration of aggressive therapies and end-of-life care.

An alternative to combined end points is the use of hierarchical end points based on ranking of events. This approach is designed to recognize that not all end points are of equal importance. In this type of scheme, all patients in a CER cohort are ranked based on a prespecified hierarchy of events. For example, time to death is ranked at the bottom, then time to hospitalization next, and so forth. The primary analysis in this type of analysis is a nonparametric comparison of the ranks between those patients receiving one intervention compared with those receiving another. Rank end points are believed to be more difficult to interpret and have rarely been used in CER. The advantages and disadvantages of global rank end points for trials of mechanical cardiac support devices and acute heart failure have been reviewed in detail.[67,68]

Statistically, the use of composites increases the total event rate and therefore may increase statistical power. However, composite end points increase statistical power only if the intervention has an effect on multiple aspects of the composite.[69] Combining end points may avoid statistical problems inherent to the individual assessment of nonmortality end points within a population of patients experiencing a high absolute death rate. Patients who die are no longer at risk for other events. If deaths are excluded (for logistic regression) or censored (for time-dependent analyses), an important subpopulation is effectively removed from the analysis. Therefore, most analyses of rehospitalization assess the combined end point of death or rehospitalization for these reasons.

CONSIDERATIONS FOR FUTURE END-POINT DESIGN

The discussion earlier helps provide general principles to guide future CER end-point selection (**Box 1**). First and foremost, CER must focus on measures of clinical importance, assessed over a reasonable duration of follow-up. Therefore, greater prospective capture of patient-reported health status and resource use, in addition to mortality, is essential to realize the full potential of CER. In addition, standardization and validation of end-point measures is critical for all types of heart-failure research. Creating a consensus on the use of consistent end points across studies (eg, all-cause mortality and rehospitalization, and

---

Box 1
Key considerations for an ideal CER end point

1. Measures something of clinical value (ie, relates to patients feeling better or living longer, or saves resources)

2. Simple to obtain

3. Easy to interpret

4. Objective, validated, and accurate

5. Accounts for the totality of patient experience, or combines multiple domains to capture important outcomes

6. Standardized between studies to allow for comparisons

the MLwHF or KCCQ to measure patient-reported health status outcomes) is critically important so that CER analyses can compare similar outcomes across studies. The fundamental purpose of CER (to compare various therapies) inherently requires that the same end points are being collected in a standardized and reproducible way. The promise of health information technology may bring more detailed clinical data capture, the ability to standardize data capture across health care systems and beyond, and even the ability to prospectively block randomize patients in routine care to various interventions for comparison. Current electronic health record companies have not sought to harmonize their clinical data elements or to support the export of these data to common databases, impeding the potential of CER using these methods.

SUMMARY

CER for heart failure continues to evolve, including its assessment of end points. Reliance on surrogate end points is unacceptable as a means of definitively establishing comparisons of clinical effectiveness. CER needs to focus on measures that clearly reflect clinical effectiveness and safety, not just survival but also standardized assessments of health status and detailed resource utilization, and it must do so in a standardized way to allow for comparison. This strategy almost certainly requires increased reliance on prospective studies with proactive end-point capture, preferably in the setting of randomized allocation of the interventions being compared.

ACKNOWLEDGMENTS

Dr. Allen was supported by grant 5K23HL105896 from the National Heart, Lung, and Blood Institute of the National Institutes of Health.

REFERENCES

1. Hunt SA, Abraham WT, Chin MH, et al. 2009 focused update incorporated into the ACC/AHA 2005 Guidelines for the Diagnosis and Management of Heart Failure in Adults: a report of the American College of Cardiology Foundation/American Heart Association Task Force on Practice Guidelines: developed in collaboration with the International Society for Heart and Lung Transplantation. Circulation 2009;119(14):e391–479.
2. Dickstein K, Cohen-Solal A, Filippatos G, et al. ESC guidelines for the diagnosis and treatment of acute and chronic heart failure 2008: the Task Force for the Diagnosis and Treatment of Acute and Chronic Heart Failure 2008 of the European Society of Cardiology. Developed in collaboration with the Heart Failure Association of the ESC (HFA) and endorsed by the European Society of Intensive Care Medicine (ESICM). Eur Heart J 2008;29(19):2388–442.
3. Lindenfeld J, Albert NM, Boehmer JP, et al. HFSA 2010 comprehensive heart failure practice guideline. J Card Fail 2010;16(6):e1–194.
4. Roger VL, Go AS, Lloyd-Jones DM, et al. Heart disease and stroke statistics–2011 update: a report from the American Heart Association. Circulation 2011;123(6):e240.
5. Allen LA, O'Connor CM. Management of acute decompensated heart failure. CMAJ 2007;176(6):797–805.
6. Paulus WJ, van Ballegoij JJ. Treatment of heart failure with normal ejection fraction: an inconvenient truth! J Am Coll Cardiol 2010;55(6):526–37.
7. Goodlin SJ, Hauptman PJ, Arnold R, et al. Consensus statement: palliative and supportive care in advanced heart failure. J Card Fail 2004; 10(3):200–9.
8. Stewart S, MacIntyre K, Hole DJ, et al. More 'malignant' than cancer? Five-year survival following a first admission for heart failure. Eur J Heart Fail 2001; 3(3):315–22.
9. Yusuf S, Negassa A. Choice of clinical outcomes in randomized trials of heart failure therapies: disease-specific or overall outcomes? Am Heart J 2002; 143(1):22–8.
10. Hohnloser SH, Kuck KH, Dorian P, et al. Prophylactic use of an implantable cardioverter-defibrillator after acute myocardial infarction. N Engl J Med 2004; 351(24):2481–8.
11. O'Connor CM, Miller AH, Konstam MA, et al. Mode of death and cardiovascular re-hospitalization in patients admitted with acute heart failure–results from the EVEREST program. Eur Heart J 2008;(Suppl 1):59–60.
12. Carson P, Anand I, O'Connor C, et al. Mode of death in advanced heart failure: the Comparison of Medical, Pacing, and Defibrillation Therapies in Heart Failure (COMPANION) trial. J Am Coll Cardiol 2005;46(12):2329–34.
13. Solomon SD, Anavekar N, Skali H, et al. Influence of ejection fraction on cardiovascular outcomes in a broad spectrum of heart failure patients. Circulation 2005;112(24):3738–44.
14. Zile MR, Gaasch WH, Anand IS, et al. Mode of death in patients with heart failure and a preserved ejection fraction: results from the Irbesartan in Heart Failure With Preserved Ejection Fraction Study (I-Preserve) trial. Circulation 2010;121(12):1393–405.
15. Mahaffey KW, Harrington RA, Akkerhuis M, et al. Systematic adjudication of myocardial infarction end-points in an international clinical trial. Curr Control Trials Cardiovasc Med 2001;2(4):180–6.
16. Fox CS, Evans JC, Larson MG, et al. A comparison of death certificate out-of-hospital coronary heart

disease death with physician-adjudicated sudden cardiac death. Am J Cardiol 2005;95(7):856–9.

17. Lewis EF, Johnson PA, Johnson W, et al. Preferences for quality of life or survival expressed by patients with heart failure. J Heart Lung Transplant 2001; 20(9):1016–24.

18. Stevenson LW, Hellkamp AS, Leier CV, et al. Changing preferences for survival after hospitalization with advanced heart failure. J Am Coll Cardiol 2008; 52(21):1702–8.

19. Stewart GC, Brooks K, Pratibhu PP, et al. Thresholds of physical activity and life expectancy for patients considering destination ventricular assist devices. J Heart Lung Transplant 2009;28(9):863–9.

20. Spertus JA. Evolving applications for patient-centered health status measures. Circulation 2008; 118(20):2103–10.

21. The Criteria Committee of the New York Heart Association. Nomenclature and criteria for diagnosis of diseases of the heart and blood vessels. Boston: Little Brown; 1964.

22. Rafeal C, Briscoe C, Davies J, et al. Limitations of the New York Heart Association functional classification system and self-reported walking distances in chronic heart failure. Heart 2007;93(4):476–82.

23. Bennett JA, Riegel B, Bittner V, et al. Validity and reliability of the NYHA classes for measuring research outcomes in patients with cardiac disease. Heart Lung 2002;31(4):262–70.

24. Allen LA, Hernandez AF, O'Connor CM, et al. End points for clinical trials in acute heart failure syndromes. J Am Coll Cardiol 2009;53(24):2248–58.

25. Pang PS, Cleland JG, Teerlink JR, et al. A proposal to standardize dyspnoea measurement in clinical trials of acute heart failure syndromes: the need for a uniform approach. Eur Heart J 2008;29(6):816–24.

26. Mahler DA, Weinberg DH, Wells CK, et al. The measurement of dyspnea. Contents, interobserver agreement, and physiologic correlates of two new clinical indexes. Chest 1984;85(6):751–8.

27. Mahler DA, Rosiello RA, Harver A, et al. Comparison of clinical dyspnea ratings and psychophysical measurements of respiratory sensation in obstructive airway disease. Am Rev Respir Dis 1987;135(6): 1229–33.

28. Allen LA, Metra M, Milo-Cotter O, et al. Improvements in signs and symptoms during hospitalization for acute heart failure follow different patterns and depend on the measurement scales used: an international, prospective registry to evaluate the evolution of measures of disease severity in acute heart failure (MEASURE-AHF). J Card Fail 2008;14(9): 777–84.

29. Rector TS, Kubo SH, Cohn JN. Validity of the Minnesota Living with Heart Failure questionnaire as a measure of therapeutic response to enalapril or placebo. Am J Cardiol 1993;71(12):1106–7.

30. Green CP, Porter CB, Bresnahan DR, et al. Development and evaluation of the Kansas City Cardiomyopathy Questionnaire: a new health status measure for heart failure. J Am Coll Cardiol 2000;35(5): 1245–55.

31. Spertus J, Peterson E, Conard MW, et al. Monitoring clinical changes in patients with heart failure: a comparison of methods. Am Heart J 2005; 150(4):707–15.

32. Soto GE, Jones P, Weintraub WS, et al. Prognostic value of health status in patients with heart failure after acute myocardial infarction. Circulation 2004; 110(5):546–51.

33. Kosiborod M, Soto GE, Jones PG, et al. Identifying heart failure patients at high risk for near-term cardiovascular events with serial health status assessments. Circulation 2007;115(15):1975–81.

34. Heidenreich PA, Spertus JA, Jones PG, et al. Health status identifies heart failure outpatients at risk for hospitalization or death. J Am Coll Cardiol 2006; 47(4):752–6.

35. Chan PS, Soto G, Jones PG, et al. Patient health status and costs in heart failure: insights from the eplerenone post-acute myocardial infarction heart failure efficacy and survival study (EPHESUS). Circulation 2009;119(3):398–407.

36. Zuluaga MC, Guallar-Castillon P, Lopez-Garcia E, et al. Generic and disease-specific quality of life as a predictor of long-term mortality in heart failure. Eur J Heart Fail 2010;12(12):1372–8.

37. The EQ-5D: An Instrument Designed to Describe and Value Health. Available at: http://www.euroqol.org/. Accessed December 18, 2010.

38. Utility Assessment of Health Related Quality of Life. Available at: http://www.healthutilities.com/. Accessed December 18, 2010.

39. Hlatky MA, Boineau ER, Higgenbotham MB, et al. A brief self-administered questionnaire to determine function capacity (The Duke Activity Status Index). Am J Cardiol 1989;64:651–4.

40. The Short Form 36. Available at: http://www.sf-36.org/. Accessed December 18, 2010.

41. Spertus JA, Tooley J, Jones P, et al. Expanding the outcomes in clinical trials of heart failure: the quality of life and economic components of EPHESUS (EPlerenone's neuroHormonal Efficacy and SUrvival Study). Am Heart J 2002;143(4):636–42.

42. Von Neumann J, Morgenstern O. Theory of games and economic behavior. 1st edition. Princeton (NJ): Princeton University Press; 1944.

43. Torrance GW, Feeny D. Utilities and quality-adjusted life years. Int J Technol Assess Health Care 1989; 5(4):559–75.

44. Torrance GW. Utility approach to measuring health-related quality of life. J Chronic Dis 1987;40(6):593–603.

45. Porter ME. What is value in health care? N Engl J Med 2010;363(26):2477–81.

46. Pearson SD, Rawlins MD. Quality, innovation, and value for money: NICE and the British National Health Service. JAMA 2005;294(20):2618–22.

47. Weinstein MC, Skinner JA. Comparative effectiveness and health care spending–implications for reform. N Engl J Med 2010;362(5):460–5.

48. Liao L, Allen LA, Whellan DJ. Economic burden of heart failure in the elderly. Pharmacoeconomics 2008;26(6):447–62.

49. Blair JE, Zannad F, Konstam MA, et al. Continental differences in clinical characteristics, management, and outcomes in patients hospitalized with worsening heart failure results from the EVEREST (Efficacy of Vasopressin Antagonism in Heart Failure: outcome Study with Tolvaptan) program. J Am Coll Cardiol 2008;52(20):1640–8.

50. Piaggio G, Elbourne DR, Altman DG, et al. Reporting of noninferiority and equivalence randomized trials: an extension of the CONSORT statement. JAMA 2006;295(10):1152–60.

51. Reed SD, Anstrom KJ, Seils DM, et al. Use of larger versus smaller drug-safety databases before regulatory approval: the trade-offs. Health Aff 2008;27(5):w360–70.

52. Prentice RL. Surrogate endpoints in clinical trials: definition and operational criteria. Stat Med 1989;8(4):431–40.

53. Bucher HC, Guyatt GH, Cook DJ, et al. Users' guides to the medical literature: XIX. Applying clinical trial results. A. How to use an article measuring the effect of an intervention on surrogate end points. Evidence-Based Medicine Working Group. JAMA 1999;282(8):771–8.

54. Sackner-Bernstein JD, Kowalski M, Fox M, et al. Short-term risk of death after treatment with nesiritide for decompensated heart failure: a pooled analysis of randomized controlled trials. JAMA 2005;293(15):1900–5.

55. Gerstein HC, Miller ME, Byington RP, et al. Effects of intensive glucose lowering in type 2 diabetes. N Engl J Med 2008;358(24):2545–59.

56. Nissen SE, Wolski K. Effect of rosiglitazone on the risk of myocardial infarction and death from cardiovascular causes. N Engl J Med 2007;356(24):2457–71.

57. Kastelein JJ, Akdim F, Stroes ES, et al. Simvastatin with or without ezetimibe in familial hypercholesterolemia. N Engl J Med 2008;358(14):1431–43.

58. Barter PJ, Caulfield M, Eriksson M, et al. Effects of torcetrapib in patients at high risk for coronary events. N Engl J Med 2007;357(21):2109–22.

59. Jones RH, Velazquez EJ, Michler RE, et al. Coronary bypass surgery with or without surgical ventricular reconstruction. N Engl J Med 2009;360(17):1705–17.

60. Publication Committee for the VMAC Investigators (Vasodilatation in the Management of Acute CHF). Intravenous nesiritide vs nitroglycerin for treatment of decompensated congestive heart failure: a randomized controlled trial. JAMA 2002;287(12):1531–40.

61. Hernandez AF, O'Connor CM, Starling RC, et al. Rationale and design of the Acute Study of Clinical Effectiveness of Nesiritide in Decompensated Heart Failure Trial (ASCEND-HF). Am Heart J 2009;157(2):271–7.

62. Mebazaa A, Nieminen MS, Packer M, et al. Levosimendan vs dobutamine for patients with acute decompensated heart failure: the SURVIVE Randomized Trial. JAMA 2007;297(17):1883–91.

63. Packer M. Randomized multicenter evaluation of intravenous levosimendan efficacy versus placebo in the short-term treatment of decompensated heart failure study (REVIVE-2). Paper presented at: Proceedings of the American Heart Association Scientific Sessions, Dallas, November 13–16, 2005.

64. Ronco C, Haapio M, House AA, et al. Cardiorenal syndrome. J Am Coll Cardiol 2008;52(19):1527–39.

65. Massie BM, O'Connor CM, Metra M, et al. Rolofylline, an adenosine A1-receptor antagonist, in acute heart failure. N Engl J Med 2010;363(15):1419–28.

66. Binanay C, Califf RM, Hasselblad V, et al. Evaluation study of congestive heart failure and pulmonary artery catheterization effectiveness: the ESCAPE trial. JAMA 2005;294(13):1625–33.

67. Felker GM, Anstrom KJ, Rogers JG. A global ranking approach to end points in trials of mechanical circulatory support devices. J Card Fail 2008;14(5):368–72.

68. Felker GM, Maisel AS. Development of therapeutics for heart failure: a global rank end point for clinical trials of acute heart failure. Circ Heart Fail 2010;3:643–6.

69. Ferreira-Gonzalez I, Busse JW, Heels-Ansdell D, et al. Problems with use of composite end points in cardiovascular trials: systematic review of randomised controlled trials. BMJ 2007;334(7597):786.

Epidemiologic and Statistical Methods for Comparative Effectiveness Research

Mark A. Hlatky, MD[a],*,
Wolfgang C. Winkelmayer, MD, MPH, ScD[b],
Soko Setoguchi, MD, DrPH[c]

KEYWORDS

- Comparative effectiveness research • Randomized trials • Observational data • Statistical methods
- Epidemiologic methods

KEY POINTS

- Methods for observational comparative effectiveness research are evolving in response to the widespread availability of data from clinical registries, electronic health records, and administrative databases.
- To conduct valid observational studies evaluating the effect of therapies in unselected populations treated in routine practice, researchers need to understand the strengths and limitations of rigorous design options and statistical methods and use them appropriately.

Comparative effectiveness research (CER) seeks to "compare the benefits and harms of alternative methods to prevent, diagnose, treat and monitor a clinical condition or to improve the delivery of care."[1] This broad scope can only be addressed by a diversified research portfolio that encompasses many types of studies, including randomized trials, observational studies, simulation models, and meta-analyses.[2] Although each of these designs has methodologic issues, observational studies to compare treatments have methodologic challenges that threaten the internal validity of their results.[3,4] This article reviews several approaches to the analysis of observational data that are in common use, or that may have promise even though they are not yet often applied. As a starting point, the analysis of randomized trials is reviewed, because many of the observational data analysis methods seek to emulate some key features of randomized trials.

RANDOMIZED TRIALS

The randomized clinical trial (RCT) is the benchmark for research quality against which all other study designs are compared. What aspects of the RCT make it the reference standard for quality? Many of the strengths of an RCT flow from the fact that it is an experiment, and the procedures to be followed in recruitment of patients, data collection, intervention, outcomes, and analyses are determined in advance by investigators. The types of patients to be enrolled are prespecified by inclusion and exclusion criteria, and suitable clinical centers are enlisted. The important pieces of information about study patients are identified at the outset, and data forms are designed to collect this essential information. Procedure manuals are written to standardize data collection, and the optimum treatment regimens are identified and applied uniformly and expertly. All patients are followed closely, and predetermined endpoint data

[a] Department of Health Research and Policy, Department of Medicine, Stanford University School of Medicine, Stanford, CA, USA; [b] Department of Medicine, Stanford University School of Medicine, Stanford, CA, USA; [c] Department of Medicine, Duke University Medical Center, Durham, NC, USA
* Corresponding author. Stanford University School of Medicine, HRP Redwood Building, Room T150, 259 Campus Drive, Stanford, CA 94305–5405.
E-mail address: hlatky@stanford.edu

Heart Failure Clin 9 (2013) 29–36
http://dx.doi.org/10.1016/j.hfc.2012.09.007
1551-7136/13/$ – see front matter © 2013 Elsevier Inc. All rights reserved.

are collected completely. Finally, the data are analyzed according to a prespecified plan to test study hypotheses. It is readily apparent from this litany that a major reason RCTs are so highly regarded is the care and planning that goes into every step of this process. It is also apparent that most of these same strengths are not specific to RCTs, and could be applied to other research studies, such as high-quality clinical data registries.

The sine qua non of the RCT is that treatment is assigned based on the value of a random number (a coin flip) rather than by the choice of the patient or treating physician. This crucial step means that patients assigned to alternative treatments are equivalent at the start of the study in all respects, within the play of chance. If the number of patients is "large," it is very unlikely that any baseline characteristic will be seriously imbalanced between the treatment groups. For instance, if there are 20 patients with a particular characteristic, a 50:50 randomization might lead to as many as 5 of these patients in one group and 15 in the other, but with 200 patients a split more extreme than 85/115 is unlikely, and for 1000 patients a split more extreme than 468/532 is unlikely. Certain procedures, such as block randomization or adaptive randomization, can further reduce the likelihood that certain key characteristics are unbalanced among treatment groups.

Although the randomization process ensures balance between the study patient groups at baseline, differences between groups may develop after randomization in background therapy, frequency of monitoring, and so forth that could affect subsequent outcomes. Randomized trials use protocols to minimize postrandomization differences in treatment or monitoring between randomly assigned groups. Blinding is a key principle that should ensure that neither the patient nor the treating physician becomes aware of the actual exposure and change their behavior in response. Clearly, it is impossible to blind for certain exposures. An important third blinding mechanism is the independent adjudication of key study outcomes of specialists that remain unaware of each patient's exposure status.

The statistical analysis of RCTs relies on the intention-to-treat principle to maintain the benefits of random assignment and avoid bias introduced by informative censoring and crossover of treatments. Thus, even if some patients assigned to Treatment A do not take it, or cross over to alternative Treatment B, their outcomes are attributed to Treatment A in the data analysis.

For all these reasons, RCTs are considered to have the highest internal validity and trials alone are considered to be capable of producing the highest level of evidence. A frequent downside of RCTs, however, is the highly selected nature of the enrolled subjects, which may limit the generalizability of the findings to the more general population of interest, or to specific subgroups of patients. In addition, trials are usually powered to detect important differences in desired outcomes, but may not be sufficiently large to compare the safety of the comparators of interest.

DATA QUALITY

Unlike RCTs, treatment in observational studies is not determined by randomization but by clinical or nonclinical reasons (indications). Confounding by indication and selection bias are the biggest threats to the internal validity of observational CER, and epidemiologic and statistical methods are needed to minimize their effects on study results. The most basic and important way to strengthen the validity of observational CER is to use high-quality data about the patients, their treatment, and their subsequent outcomes.

The quality of data should be assessed by at least three aspects: (1) kinds of information (types of variables); (2) accuracy of that information (specificity and sensitivity); and (3) amount of information (completeness). A clinical registry of patients with heart failure could, for instance, collect data using standardized forms and data definitions, which would ensure that the key information about the patients (especially about their heart failure characteristics and other cardiovascular comorbidities) is available for analysis. However, the completeness and accuracy of information can vary considerably depending on the method of collection and incentives of providers. Also, the follow-up information in many clinical registries is often short (mostly up to 6 months) and incomplete. Claims data, such as Medicare Part A, B, and D files, provide longitudinal data on a large real world representative population. For major clinical outcomes, such as hospitalizations and death, claims data provide accurate and complete information. However, billing diagnoses submitted to Medicare or private insurers are less accurate than diagnoses in registries or electronic health records. Furthermore, claims data do not contain important clinical information, such as New York Heart Association functional class; findings from the physical examination; or the results of laboratory or imaging examinations (eg, ejection fraction). Solutions to overcome limitations of various data sources include linking existing databases (eg, link a registry with claims data, link electronic health records or laboratory records to claims data)[5,6] and collecting additional information to supplement existing databases by surveying patients or reviewing medical records (a more comprehensive review is provided elsewhere in this issue).

NEW-USER DESIGNS

Another advantage of randomized trials is that "time zero" is well defined by the date of randomization, and treatments are initiated at "time zero." The paramount importance of mimicking this design in observational CER, where it is called "new-user design," has long been recognized.[7] Inclusion of patients who have been on a treatment for some time before "time zero" for a study may lead to biased associations. Prevalent users (patients who started a drug and remained on a drug) are a selected subset, because patients who cannot tolerate the drug, patients who develop complications, and patients who are not adherent have all dropped out, and the remaining users are more likely to be adherent, have favorable health behaviors, and be tolerant of the study drug. Also, including prevalent users in a treatment group can underestimate the event rate in the treatment group if events early in the course of treatment are not captured. Comparing prevalent users with other patients is likely to give a biased picture of the treatment's safety and efficacy.

The new-user design attempts to minimize these problems by identifying a cohort of patients who are newly started on a treatment.[7] The implementation of the design requires a look-back period of some duration (typically 6–12 months in claims data) to ensure that the patients were previously not on a treatment of interest. A related strategy is to identify patients with new onset of the disease who are then started on the study drug, because newly diagnosed individuals are unlikely to have been previously treated. For example, patients with new onset of heart failure may be less likely to have been treated with multiple prior drug regiments, and more likely to be new users of heart failure drugs. However, many drugs used to treat heart failure can also be used to treat hypertension (eg, angiotensin-converting enzyme inhibitors, β-blockers) or other cardiac conditions (eg, digoxin for atrial fibrillation), so merely identifying patients with new-onset heart failure does not necessarily identify new users of these drugs. By contrast, patients with newly diagnosed diabetes are most unlikely to have been treated previously with metformin, proglitazone, or insulin, because these drugs are used solely to treat diabetes.

The new-user design is strongly recommended to control biases introduced by including prevalent users (survivor bias and selection bias), but in and of itself does not fully control for confounding bias. After a suitable cohort of new users is identified, other epidemiologic and statistical techniques are still needed to control for confounding, especially for confounding by indication.

Related to the new-user design is the concept of studying only "treatment eligible" patients. For example, if one wished to compare two drugs, one of which is contraindicated in patients with chronic kidney disease, it would bias the results of a comparison study to include any patients with chronic kidney disease. The patients with chronic kidney disease are likely to have worse outcomes than other patients, and if they were predominantly treated with one drug, their worse outcomes would bias the study results against that drug. So, when comparing two drugs, patients with contraindications to one or the other drug are best excluded, much as they would be in a randomized trial of the two drugs. Furthermore, there is no clinical question about which drug to choose when one of the drugs is contraindicated.

OVERVIEW OF STATISTICAL METHODS TO CONTROL CONFOUNDING

Confounding and selection bias are the biggest threats to the validity in observational CER. In observational CER studies, it is necessary to use epidemiologic and statistical methods that attempt to achieve the balance in prognostic characteristics of patients to avoid confounding without randomization.[8] Various methods exist to control for potential confounding (**Fig. 1**). Although the importance of classic design and methods, such as restriction or stratification, should not be underestimated, this article focuses on the concept and use of methods that are more recent and increasing in their popularity. First discussed are methods to adjust for measured confounding: propensity score-based approaches and marginal structural models as representatives of so-called causal methods. Next reviewed are the concept and use of instrumental variable (IV) analysis as a method to control for measured and unmeasured confounding and the importance of sensitivity analyses in assessment of unmeasured confounding.

PROPENSITY SCORES

In the real world, treatments are determined by physicians and patients based on various factors including patient characteristics, clinical

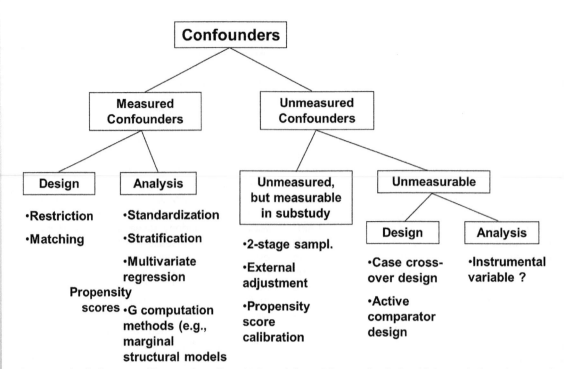

Fig. 1. Methods for controlling confounding. (*Adapted from* Schneeweiss S. Sensitivity analysis and external adjustment for unmeasured confounders in epidemiologic database studies of therapeutics. Pharmacoepidemiol Drug Saf 2006;15(5):291–303; with permission.)

presentations, availability of treatment options, and patients' and physicians' preferences, but not by randomization. When assessing the effect of treatments, controlling for confounding is essential because these factors influencing the choice of treatments often affect the outcome of interest. The propensity score method attempts to control for confounding by balancing the factors influencing the treatment choice. The first step for propensity score analysis is to develop a model predicting the treatment based on measured factors (covariates), which yields a probability that any individual patient will receive Treatment A instead of Treatment B. This exposure propensity score model is typically developed using a multivariable logistic regression modeling in which the dependent variable is a dichotomous variable indicating the received treatment, and the independent (predictor) variables are a set of variables for measured patient characteristics and other factors potentially influencing the treatment choice:

$$P(T_{ij}) = f(X_i, Y_j)$$

where

T_{ij} = the treatment given to patient "i" by; provider "j"

X_i = patient-level characteristics

Y_j = provider-level characteristics

For instance, the treatment might be prescribed to a patient with heart failure on the basis of the patient's age, gender, cause of heart failure, functional class, left ventricular ejection fraction, and QRS duration on the electrocardiogram. An exposure propensity score model estimates a set of regression coefficients for all included variables for the study population. Because each patient's characteristics are (ideally) known ("covariate vector"), this information can then be combined with the regression coefficients to calculate each patient's predicted probability of receiving Treatment A, which is the propensity score. Because it is a probability, the propensity score is bound by [0, 1].

The second step of propensity score analysis, after the propensity score is estimated, is to achieve a balance in the propensity scores between the two treatment groups (Treatment A and B in this example). Three different approaches based on propensity scores are currently used and capable of achieving balanced characteristics between treatment groups (**Box 1**) and controversy remains about the optimal approach. One key prerequisite in selecting and justifying an optimal approach is to compare the distribution of estimated propensity scores between patients who received Treatment A and Treatment B. In the unlikely event that these two distributions have no or very little overlap (indicated by almost perfect predictive capability of the model

Box 1	
Methods for propensity score adjustment	
Matching	Match on the value of propensity score. The most commonly used matching method is greedy matching.
Strafitification	Stratify by quintiles ~ deciles of propensity score. Can be done with or without trimming.
Propensity score adjustment in outcome regression model	Include propensity score as independent variable in a regression outcome model. Propensity score can be included as a continuous variables or indicator variables for quintiles or deciles. Can be done with or without trimming.
Trimming	Exclude patients with extreme values for propensity scores to avoid inclusion of nonoverlapping or less overlapping patients.

[eg, measured by a concordance (c) statistic of the exposure propensity score model very close to 1]), the conclusion would be that patients getting the alternative treatments are so completely different that they may not be validly compared. For example, if all the men got Treatment A and all the women got Treatment B, it would be impossible to disentangle the effects on outcome of treatment and of gender.

As long as the distributions of propensity scores overlap, Treatment A might be compared with Treatment B by propensity score matching, stratification, or direct adjustment in regression analysis, with or without trimming (see **Box 1**). Matching patients on propensity score is the method suggested by Rubin[8] and ensures that nonoverlapping patients are excluded from the analyses. This method also has intuitive appeal and face validity. There are various algorithms for matching groups of patients on propensity score that range from selecting an exact match to closest match with various fineness of the caliper. The goal of propensity score analyses is to achieve the balance in measured covariates in the two treatment groups. By matching on propensity score, the study

population has similar distribution of measured covariates, which is seen in two groups with random treatment assignment. However, it is crucial to recognize that propensity score analysis, in theory and in general, only achieves balance for measured factors that are included in the propensity score model, whereas randomization achieves balance for measured and unmeasured factors. Other propensity score–based approaches can be thought of as extensions of the matching process by relaxing the matching caliper (see **Box 1**). Stratification on propensity score involves dividing the entire population into quintiles (or deciles) of propensity score, and within each quintile comparing the outcomes of patients who received Treatment A with the outcomes of patients who received Treatment B. The patients in each quintile should all have sufficiently "similar" propensity scores, even though they were not matched.

Finally, propensity scores can be used as independent predictor variables in outcome models (typically a Cox or logistic model) to adjust for the propensity to receive Treatment A versus Treatment B.

The stratification and regression approaches to using the propensity score have been criticized for including patients in the tails of the distribution of scores who are extremely unlikely to receive the alternate therapy and have no "match." This criticism can be overcome to some extent by restricting the analysis to patients who fall within the overlapping regions of the distribution of propensity scores (ie, by trimming the distribution, then comparing outcomes of the remaining patients) (see **Box 1**).[9]

Theoretically, the propensity score method has the advantage of reducing all the factors affecting treatment decisions into a single number. When comparing the results from multivariable models with propensity score adjusted models in studies that reported both, no meaningful differences in effect estimates were observed in almost all studies,[10,11] suggesting that propensity score adjustment adds little compared with using traditional multivariable adjustment for the same factors in the outcome model. Only in situations where outcomes are too scarce for adjustment of all relevant variables in a multivariable model because of the risk of model overfitting, propensity scores may provide a methodologic alternative. In addition to its use in situations of rare outcomes, another advantage of propensity score approach over traditional multivariate analyses is the possibility to remove extreme cases of treatment assignment from the dataset. Specifically, it is desirable to remove patients that have extremely low propensity for receiving Treatment A, but still received it, or patients with extremely high propensity for Treatment A, who still received Treatment B. These individuals usually reside in the area of nonoverlap of the two propensity score distributions. Frequently, these patients also often have either particularly bad or particularly good prognosis, which makes them influential observations. Propensity matching is an excellent method to eliminate such observations, as is "trimming," removal of observations in the extremes of the propensity score distributions or the areas of nonoverlap. Using either of these methods increases internal validity. There may be some loss of external validity, however, but this is often a useful compromise.

Once again, the fundamental limitation to any propensity score approach is that the method does not adjust for unmeasured confounding. Some factors that were important in the treatment decision and were associated with the outcome of interest may not have been recorded in the data, and hence cannot be included in the propensity score model and cannot be adjusted. For instance, a clinician's gestalt of patients who "look older than their stated age" or who seem to have "poor protoplasm" may be important in the choice of treatment and the patient's subsequent outcome. Even well-designed heart failure registries do not capture this kind of clinician's impression, so residual confounding caused by this unmeasured factor would remain even after exact matching on propensity score. Again, this problem of residual confounding caused by unmeasured factors does not occur in a randomized trial, because patients with "poor protoplasm" who are randomized will still be equally likely to be assigned to Treatment A or Treatment B.

MARGINAL STRUCTURAL MODELS

Heart failure can be treated with devices and procedures (eg, cardiac surgery) that are applied once and have long-lasting effects. These exposures are relatively straightforward to measure. In contrast, pharmacologic treatments for heart failure are supposed to be chronic treatment regimens, but they may be changed over time or discontinued because of side effects or poor adherence. It is much more complicated to assess the effectiveness of these time-varying treatments, because accurate identification of exposure and assessment and adjustment of time-varying confounding are challenging. To adjust for time-varying confounding, highly sophisticated approaches have been developed.

Marginal structural models, a member of the family of g-estimation methods, were initially developed to assess the efficacy of antiretroviral treatment for AIDS.[12] The HIV treatment regimens were often changed in response to results of laboratory tests, such as CD4 cell counts, that were also prognostic markers and therefore became confounders that were time-varying in studies assessing the effectiveness of HIV treatment regimen. In this situation, the probability of treatment at any time t_i depended on the patient's condition at time t_i, and on prior treatment at time t_{i-1}. In a marginal structural model, the outcomes of patients who receive treatment A at time t_i are weighted by the inverse probability that they received Treatment A, and the outcomes of patients who received Treatment B are weighted by the inverse probability of receiving Treatment B (if there are only two alternatives $P_i[B] = 1 - P_i[A]$). The outcomes of Treatment A and B are then compared in a weighted model. Note that the probability of receiving a given treatment is akin to a propensity score, although these probabilities are used in the analysis as weights.

Marginal structural models are in principle a powerful tool for dissecting the effect of treatments that vary over time, where time-varying confounding threatens the internal validity, such as drugs or monitoring strategies. These models depart from the "intention-to-treat" paradigm for analyzing the effects of drug treatment in an RCT, however, because periods of time when a patient is off Treatment A are not counted against Treatment A in a marginal structural model, but they are in an RCT analyzed under the intention-to-treat principle. The extension of the method can be used to model and adjust for informative censoring or discontinuation. Despite the attractiveness of the idea and extensive research on the method, it has not been used extensively.[13] One of the reasons and also the biggest challenge in operationalizing and effectively making use of the method is lack of detailed data on the time-varying exposure (treatment) and time-varying confounders in most data sources. Without precise data on the exposure and confounders that are measured in a time-varying manner, the method does add beyond other traditional methods. In addition, the method can still not account for any confounders, time-dependent or not, which are unrecorded.

INSTRUMENTAL VARIABLES

Economists rarely do experimental studies and consequently have developed many powerful tools to analyze observational data and draw causal inferences. Health economists have applied some of these econometric techniques to compare the effect of treatments on clinical outcomes. IV methods are particularly attractive for this purpose. The distinct characteristics of the IV method, as opposed to propensity scoring and marginal structural models, is its theoretical ability to adjust for unmeasured confounding.[14,15] The method has been applied in several prominent studies in cardiovascular medicine.[16,17]

Conceptually, an "instrument" is a variable that predicts the treatment used, and does not directly or indirectly affect subsequent outcome (ie, is only correlated with outcome to the extent that it is correlated with choice of treatment). Randomization is actually an example of a perfect "instrument": it is highly correlated with choice of treatment, and only affects outcome through the choice of treatment, not by itself. Identification of a good instrument is not straightforward, however, and usually requires a clever insight into the specific treatment at hand. For instance, formulary committees at different hospitals may select different drugs for use in patients with heart failure, facilitating observational comparisons among similar patient populations.[18] Some tests and procedures may be available on weekdays but not on weekends, leading to different management of otherwise similar patients admitted on different days of the week. A new therapy may be introduced on a certain date, and patients treated before that date could not receive it, whereas patients treated later could receive the new therapy. Identification of such natural experiments can be exploited to compare treatment outcomes even though patients were not randomized.

If a suitable instrument can be found, an IV analysis basically compares patients who have different exposures to the instrument, but are otherwise similar:

$$O(X_i) = f(X_i, IV_i)$$

where

X_i = patients characteristics known to affect outcome, and

IV_i = value of the instrumental variable for patient "i"

If the IV shifts 20% of patients from Treatment A to Treatment B and outcomes change by 2%, the IV approach would estimate that a 100% shift from Treatment A to Treatment B would lead to a 10% change in outcome. This estimate of the treatment effect can be sharpened by additional statistical controls for differences in baseline clinical characteristics.

The major limitation of the IV approach is the difficulty in identifying a suitable instrument, because good "natural experiments" are haphazard. If the instrument is weak and shifts in treatment are very small (eg, from 40% use to 42% use of a drug or device), it is less convincing that any outcome differences are truly because of differences in treatment, and not due to differences in other clinical factors. Also, even if a suitable or reasonable instrument can be identified, the assumptions that are necessary for the IV to be valid cannot be tested or validated fully. It is usually possible to judge whether observed baseline characteristics are balanced across levels of the instrument. If that is the case, one may be assured that the instrument may also balance unobserved characteristics. If the instrument does not balance observed characteristics, one can certainly include such observed information in formal IV analysis; however, it is less plausible that unobserved characteristics are balanced across levels of the instrument. The judgment on the validity of the IV analysis will be left to theoretical and substantive discussion.

SUMMARY

Observational methods are evolving in response to the widespread availability of data from clinical registries, electronic health records, and administrative databases. These approaches will never eliminate the need for randomized trials, but clearly have a role in evaluating the effect of therapies in unselected populations treated in routine practice.

REFERENCES

1. Institute of Medicine. Initial national priorities for comparative effectiveness research. Washington: The National Academies Press; 2009.
2. Hlatky MA, Douglas PS, Cook NL, et al. Future directions for cardiovascular disease comparative effectiveness research. Report of a workshop sponsored by the National Heart, Lung, and Blood Institute. J Am Coll Cardiol 2012;60:569–80.
3. Normand SL. Some old and some new statistical tools for outcomes research. Circulation 2008;118:872–84.
4. Johnson ML, Crown W, Martin BC, et al. Good research practices for comparative effectiveness research: analytic methods to improve causal inference from nonrandomized studies of treatment effects using secondary data sources: the ISPOR Good Research Practices for Retrospective Database Analysis Task Force Report–Part III. Value Health 2009;12:1062–73.
5. Setoguchi S, Glynn RJ, Avorn J, et al. Statins and the risk of lung, breast, and colorectal cancer in the elderly. Circulation 2007;115:27–33.
6. Hammill BG, Hernandez AF, Peterson ED, et al. Linking inpatient clinical registry data to Medicare claims

data using indirect identifiers. Am Heart J 2009;157: 995–1000.

7. Ray WA. Evaluating medication effects outside of clinical trials: new-user designs. Am J Epidemiol 2003;158:915–20.

8. Rubin DB. The design versus the analysis of observational studies for causal effects: parallels with the design of randomized trials. Stat Med 2007;26:20–36.

9. Kurth T, Walker AM, Glynn RJ, et al. Results of multivariable logistic regression, propensity matching, propensity adjustment, and propensity-based weighting under conditions of nonuniform effect. Am J Epidemiol 2006;163:262–70.

10. Shah BR, Laupacis A, Hux JE, et al. Propensity score methods gave similar results to traditional regression modeling in observational studies: a systematic review. J Clin Epidemiol 2005;58:550–9.

11. Stürmer T, Joshi M, Glynn RJ, et al. A review of the application of propensity score methods yielded increasing use, advantages in specific settings, but not substantially different estimates compared with conventional multivariable methods. J Clin Epidemiol 2006;59:437–47.

12. Robins JM, Hernán MA, Brumback B. Marginal structural models and causal inference in epidemiology. Epidemiology 2000;11:550–60.

13. Mehrotra R, Chiu YW, Kalantar-Zadeh K, et al. Similar outcomes with hemodialysis and peritoneal dialysis in patients with end-stage renal disease. Arch Intern Med 2011;171:110–8.

14. Rassen JA, Brookhart MA, Glynn RJ, et al. Instrumental variables I: instrumental variables exploit natural variation in nonexperimental data to estimate causal relationships. J Clin Epidemiol 2009;62: 1226–32.

15. Brookhart MA, Rassen JA, Schneeweiss S. Instrumental variable methods in comparative safety and effectiveness research. Effective health care research report No. 22 (Prepared by Brigham and Women's Hospital DEcIDE Center Under Contract No. 290-2005-00161 T03). Rockville (MD): Agency for Healthcare Research and Quality; 2010. Available at: http://effectivehealthcare.ahrq.gov/reports/final.cfm. Accessed July 9, 2011.

16. McClellan M, McNeil BJ, Newhouse JP. Does more intensive treatment of acute myocardial infarction in the elderly reduce mortality? Analysis using instrumental variables. JAMA 1994;272:859–66.

17. Stukel TA, Fisher ES, Wennberg DE, et al. Analysis of observational studies in the presence of treatment selection bias: effects of invasive cardiac management on AMI survival using propensity score and instrumental variable methods. JAMA 2007;297:278–85.

18. Johnston SC, Henneman T, McCulloch CE, et al. Modeling treatment effects on binary outcomes with grouped-treatment variables and individual covariates. Am J Epidemiol 2002;156:753–60.

Comparative Effectiveness Research
Drug-Drug Comparisons in Heart Failure

Emil L. Fosbol, MD, PhD

KEYWORDS

- Comparative effectiveness research • Drug-drug comparisons • Randomized clinical trials
- Heart failure

KEY POINTS

- CER offers the potential to answer many key questions about tailoring and improving the management of patients.
- One priority of CER is evaluating the translation of RCT findings into practice and evaluating the effectiveness and safety of therapies in populations and settings not included in RCTs.
- CER provides great opportunities for guiding researchers and clinicians in improving management of heart failure, which is characterized by excess morbidity, mortality, and costs.

INTRODUCTION

Randomized clinical trials (RCTs) are a primary source of evidence for clinical decision making; however, the reality is that most current treatments and decisions made in medicine are not substantiated by strong RCT evidence.[1] Even though cardiovascular medicine is one of the most evidence-based fields of medicine, only approximately 11% of clinical practice guideline recommendations are based on the highest level of evidence.[1] RCTs are time-consuming and very costly to conduct, address frequently only a narrow question and set of outcomes, and the results are often not uniformly generalizable to patients treated in typical practice settings. Hence, other sources of information are needed to complement the information derived from typical Phase III RCTs. To help fill these knowledge gaps, the American Recovery and Reinvestment Act of 2009 provided funding for advancing comparative effectiveness research (CER). CER offers the potential to answer many key questions about tailoring and improving

the management of patients, with a priority of evaluating the translation of RCT findings into practice and evaluating the effectiveness and safety of therapies in populations and settings not included in the RCTs.[2-6]

In addition, the US Food and Drug Administration launched the Sentinel Initiative in 2007 to try to address the recognized need for establishing a near "real-time" surveillance system for drug safety in the United States.[7] This need for large-scale, systematic postmarket drug surveillance underlines that not only are rigorous methods needed to detect safety signals more accurately, but that speed and precision in defining such signals after their initial detection are perhaps even more important.[7] However, no universal guidelines exist for optimally performing CER and it is extremely important to delineate the strengths and weaknesses of CER. Furthermore, it is important to determine the most appropriate role for CER using observational study designs versus when RCTs would be the best approach to address a key research question. This article outlines the strengths and weaknesses

Funding sources: Nil.
Duke Clinical Research Institute, Duke University Medical Center, 2400 Pratt Street, Room 7461, Terrace Level, Durham, NC 27705, USA
E-mail address: emil.fosbol@duke.edu

Heart Failure Clin 9 (2013) 37–47
http://dx.doi.org/10.1016/j.hfc.2012.09.008
1551-7136/13/$ – see front matter © 2013 Elsevier Inc. All rights reserved.

of drug-drug CER, with a specific focus on heart failure (HF) research, to characterize the optimal use of and approaches to CER. Although there have been important therapeutic advances in HF over the past several decades, CER provides great opportunities for guiding researchers and clinicians in improving management of this important disease characterized by excess morbidity, mortality, and costs.

DEFINITION OF DRUG-DRUG CER

Despite the recent national interest in CER, it is not entirely new, but rather is a set of methods for observational and interventional research. The Institute of Medicine committee defines CER as[8]

> ...the generation and synthesis of evidence that compares the benefits and harms of alternative methods to prevent, diagnose, treat, and monitor a clinical condition or to improve the delivery of care. The purpose of CER is to assist consumers, clinicians, purchasers, and policy makers to make informed decisions that will improve health care at both the individual and population levels.

The key words in this definition are "compares the benefits and harms of alternative methods" and "informed decisions." Hence, drug-drug CER, by definition, compares outcomes related to effectiveness or safety of individual drugs for a defined condition, population, or setting.

Overall, drug-drug comparisons would optimally answer the question of a causal link between drug A and outcomes compared with drug B (or even no drug). However, and crucial for the interpretation of drug-drug CER, observational studies can establish associations between drugs and outcomes but not a clear causal link. Relationships or associations between exposures and outcomes are the key elements of epidemiology and the terminology of CER is largely derived from traditional epidemiology. Therefore, drug-drug comparison is conceptually just the comparison of rates of outcomes between groups of patients who use different drugs for a similar indication. However, because assignment to one treatment group or the other is not random (as in an RCT), there are several concerns about other factors besides treatment exposure that could explain any observed differences in outcomes between groups. Thus, the field of CER focuses on design and analytic approaches to reduce the impact of treatment selection to allow for the least biased estimate of treatment-related effects.

METHODOLOGIC ISSUES OF DRUG-DRUG CER
Data Sources

Data sources are a crucial element in CER, and because the world of informatics is developing rapidly, the need for even more rigorously controlled data sources and better methods becomes more evident as more people gain access to large electronic datasets. A main limitation of observational CER is the nonrandom assignment of patients to different treatment groups (ie, treatment selection bias or "channeling") based on characteristics that could influence the risk of various clinical outcomes independent of the treatment itself. However, through prudent study designs, collecting data properly, and using rigorous statistical methods, the impact of bias can be minimized and interpretation can build strong associations. Large RCT datasets are often a good starting place for post hoc questions of drug-drug comparisons, but are limited by selected patient samples based on the trial's inclusion and exclusion criteria and sample sizes that are typically underpowered for evaluating safety-related outcomes. In turn, clinical registries (eg, American College of Cardiology National Cardiovascular Disease Registries) are often substantially larger in size but have limitations including inclusion of only volunteer institutions, have selected data about a specific episode of care or procedure, and typically are cross-sectional in nature.

To address some of these issues, additional efforts have been made for selected clinical registries to link with administrative databases (eg, Medicare claims, National Death Index), which can provide longitudinal data on mortality, hospitalizations, comorbidity, procedures, and in selected patients drug prescription claims.[9] This linkage facilitates CER studies over a longer time horizon for various outcomes, but existing data sources are often limited to administrative claims-based datasets that can suffer from problems in data quality and completeness, and the available population that can be linked. For example, US Center for Medicare and Medicaid Services data are primarily restricted to older patients (age ≥ 65 years) who qualified for Medicare insurance, fee-for-service beneficiaries, the years of data available for prescription drug data are still limited, and data are only available with a significant time lag. However, the volume of Medicare prescription drug claims is increasing, which will allow for more extensive drug-drug CER studies in the future. Some European countries (eg, Denmark, Sweden, United Kingdom, The Netherlands) and also some US integrated health care delivery systems (eg, Kaiser Permanente) already have the opportunity to study drug effectiveness and safety longitudinally because they have large administrative databases including information on hospitalizations, drug prescriptions, sociodemographics, and vital status for large samples of patients and these resources have also been put to great use for conducting CER for decades. The major advantage of these resources is that the health systems are integrated and hence the data collected are comprehensive for their covered populations. Selected health systems, such as Kaiser Permanente or the Veterans Affairs, capture detailed clinical data, such as laboratory test results, other diagnostic test results, vital signs, pathology findings, and so forth. Collectively, there are many different data sources for doing drug-drug CER, but an important caveat is the way in which the data are used and for what purpose. Definitions of the study population, exposures, outcomes, and relevant covariates are extremely important, along with the ability to assess these key factors properly within different data sources when planning for rigorous CER studies.

Defining Drug Exposure

Drug exposure can be defined in many different ways depending on the level of detail and comprehensiveness of data for individual drugs in a specific data source. Clinical trial datasets often have detailed data about relevant drug use at baseline, but longitudinal data on drug use in follow-up are often missing. Hence, the exposure definition of a certain drug (other than the possible drug tested through randomization) is frequently defined as a yes/no variable at baseline. This means that the researcher must assume full persistence of drug use after baseline, and because it is unknown who stopped treatment and when they did so, the measures of exposure can be rather crude. For drug-drug CER, it is much better to apply a study design that incorporates longitudinal drug exposure to allow more accurate assessment and timing of exposure and their relations to the occurrence of clinical outcomes during the same study period.

Drug exposure would optimally be defined daily by having pill dispensers that electronically record whether patients take the drugs as prescribed; however, this is very costly and not practical at present. Researchers must therefore rely on other methods to describe exposure in more detail longitudinally and integrate the pattern of use of the individual drug. For longitudinal studies, data from individual-level prescription claims (actual dispensing) usually serve as the mode for defining drug exposure. Depending on the patterns of drug dispensing, the setting in which it is delivered, and the outcome of interest, the drug exposure can be defined either as a dichotomous variable (treatment at a certain time: yes or no) or as a time-varying variable. For treatments of long duration with low probability of discontinuation standard exposure definitions (yes or no at baseline ~ intention-to-treat analog) may be suitable, whereas short-duration treatments are best assessed using time-varying exposure-variables (~ on treatment-analog). Time-varying exposure variables ensure that the patient is only considered exposed when he or she appears to be actually receiving the drug. By creating a "drug diary" for each patient based on prescription dispensing, longitudinal exposure can be assigned, and patients can be considered "on" or "off" treatment at different times during follow-up. This approach focuses primarily on the effects of current treatment rather than potential delayed drug-related effects, although the latter can be evaluated by applying lag effect periods to the definition of exposure. For example, the effect of amiodarone, a drug with a very long half-life, would be underestimated if the patient was considered to be nonexposed from the day of discontinuation. Amiodarone persists in the body for more than 3 months after discontinuation, and it would therefore be reasonable to add a lag effect period for this drug and define the patient as still being "exposed" for 3 months after amiodarone is discontinued.

Hence, exposure definitions depend on the question asked and the treatment setting and are important, particularly using claims data, and in longitudinal studies. Often, sensitivity analyses are needed to show several strategies to underline the robustness of the results. Overall, standard dichotomous exposure variables answer the question whether any use of drug X is related to the outcome Y (intention-to-treat analog analysis), whereas time-varying variables answer the question whether current use of drug X versus noncurrent use of X related to outcome Y (on-treatment analog analysis). These are very similar equations, but also very different in regards to the interpretation of the results. In addition, to minimize bias cause by depletion of susceptible and loss of events that occur soon after the initiation of the treatment, a new-user design by restriction to patients who initiated the exposure or comparison treatment is ideal.[10] If the drug exposure is assessed in a time-varying manner each patient has a longitudinal record of assigned drug exposure during the follow-up by linking consecutive dispensing based on dispensing dates and reported days supply. Discontinuation of treatment is also crucial and more uncertain defined by claims data compared with treatment initiation. Patients are often classified as discontinuers as soon as they fail to refill the study drug for a short period of time (eg, 7 days). Although there is no ideal way to determine this grace period,[11] a 7-day period is an exposure coding with high specificity and leads to less attenuated relative risk estimates from random misclassification of exposure,[12] but the optimal decision about the length of the grace period depends on the drug, outcome, and populations of interest.

Adherence to a therapy is often quantified by simply counting the number of patients using a specific drug at a certain point in time (ie, how many patients with HF are filling a prescription for a β-blocker after their first hospitalization for HF). Persistence is a similar measure but incorporates the function of time: persistence is supposed to quantify how many patients continue treatment with drug X over time (ie, how many HF patients are still on β-blockers 1 year after starting treatment). This is obviously a crude metric because it only incorporates two points in time (baseline and 1 year). Consequently, "medication possession ratio" is often used to quantify the percentage of the time during a certain time period that a patient is taking the drug of interest. Proportion-of-days covered is often used as a medication possession ratio and an arbitrary cut-off point at 80% is frequently used to define patients as being persistent to a treatment (ie, patients who have 80% or more of 1 year covered by β-blockers are classified as persistent to the treatment).

Another potential bias in examining drug exposure and outcomes is "immortal-time-bias," which easily occurs when comparing patients who filled a prescription for a drug X after an event with patients who did not fill a prescription after the event. When drug exposure is defined in this manner the drug-exposed individuals are effectively "immortal" until day Y, because they had to survive that long to fill their prescription. Excluding this time in the analysis introduces a bias in favor of the drug. This phenomenon is especially important when exposure is defined after an event (ie, use of drug X within 30 days of discharge from a HF hospitalization).[13–15] Immortal-time-bias can be avoided when using time-varying exposure variables or by handling follow-up time carefully in the study design.[13–15]

Defining Outcomes

Outcomes of drug-drug CER can be many but are often centered on the same key questions: are the drugs effective and are they safe? Clinical outcomes are equally crucial as exposure is for the interpretation of the results. Trials often collect and adjudicate certain prespecified outcomes as part of the protocol for a fixed time-period and hence have detailed and validated information for time-to-event analyses. Unfortunately, outcome definitions often vary between RCTs for standard endpoints[16–18] and the guidelines regarding this subject are often not followed.[16,19,20] RCT databases are suited for observational post hoc outcome analyses but are limited to per protocol analyses of captured endpoints in addition to the duration of follow-up. However, longitudinal claims-based studies (mainly using a retrospective cohort design) are not limited to certain outcomes and often the time span is longer and the population is less restrictive than in corresponding RCTs. However, a major limitation of claims-based outcome studies is that some outcomes may not be ascertained completely or accurately. Claims data are built on the payment systems for health care, so identification of outcome events (eg, diagnoses derived from hospitalizations, emergency department visits, or outpatient clinic visits) is best captured if the health care provider is paid for the care based on receiving that diagnosis. For example, hospitals are paid a large amount of money when a patient is admitted with HF, but the payment does not change whether the patient is obese, so obesity may not be recorded accurately. In addition, a comorbid condition, such as a drug allergy, is less likely to be captured because this diagnosis does not necessarily affect the care of the patient during an unrelated hospitalization and does not increase reimbursement. It is important to know the validity of the studied outcome, and sound drug-drug CER is reliant on validation studies with the calculation of specificity and positive predictive value of the method used to define the outcome in the studied population. Many regularly studied outcomes have been validated in different data sources, whereas other outcomes are studied without any information regarding the validity of the outcome (positive predictive value data are especially missing). This is an important limitation and should optimally always be done before the proper outcomes study.

Another interesting question is whether there is a delayed effect or a cumulative effect of a drug. Delayed toxicity (eg, long-term risk of cancer) is hard to assess. Delayed effects can be assessed by comparing absolute rates among users and nonusers or by performing with-in drug class comparisons, which reduces the risk of confounding by indication. Cumulative drug effects are also an interesting aspect of drug-drug CER that requires a large longitudinal database to assess accumulation of drug exposure over many years.

Defining Comparators

When the exposure of interest has been defined, it is important to define the most appropriate comparison group. In a well-executed RCT, the process of randomization balances measured and unmeasured confounders between the groups, whereas in observational drug-drug CER, balance must be achieved by careful study design and statistical analysis methods. For example, in a study of the incidence of HF among people treated with a specific chemotherapy agent, people treated with chemotherapy are distinctly different from a random sample of people not treated with chemotherapy; consequently, the relative risk of HF caused by the drug is difficult to assess. Multivariable regression analysis could potentially adjust for many of the conditions unevenly distributed, but may not be adequate depending on the covariates available and the degree of overlap in the distribution of relevant covariates. Instead of comparing users with nonusers, a study could instead compare the incidence of HF among the users of different chemotherapeutic drugs, but this approach may have limited generalizability and statistical power depending on the comparison. Another problem, however, becomes evident because different chemotherapeutics are used for different cancers. Comparing an agent used for late-stage lung cancer with an agent used for early stage colon cancer would compare both the drugs and the patients with different tumors; this important phenomenon is called confounding-by-indication. Hence, individual drugs used for similar indications would best be compared and also classes of drugs (drug-drug and class-class comparison, respectively). This is unfortunately not always possible and the researcher must use additional methodologic approaches to perform even comparisons. Such approaches include multivariable adjustment (including propensity adjusted); matching (including propensity matching); use of instrumental variables; and whether results are reproducible and maybe externally validated. The purpose of these methods is to overcome the lack of randomization and to balance the groups evenly conditional on the information that has been gathered. Propensity score matching is a sound method to balance cases and controls, but it is still important to realize that the researcher is only able to balance the groups based on the information at hand and unmeasured confounding is still a limitation to the study design. However, the number of tools in the drug-drug CER toolbox is growing and powerful when limitations are realized and best handled in the analysis.

Effectiveness Versus Safety

Effectiveness and safety are two sides of the same coin in drug-drug CER. Sound effectiveness and safety-related CER are complicated and the design of the study, particularly selection of exposure and comparator, is extremely important to assess the clinically relevant effects of a drug taken under usual care circumstances. As an example, β-blockers are core evidence-based medications for patients with HF; however, not all patients with HF get β-blockers because of a variety of reasons (side-effects, allergy, pulmonary disease, and so forth). The researcher comparing outcomes of patients prescribed a β-blocker with patients who were not prescribed a β-blocker may get a result that relates more to reasons patients were not prescribed the medication rather than the effect of the medication itself. This problem is mitigated when the study compares individual β-blockers, and assesses their effect on outcomes. Drug-drug comparisons within classes of drugs (also known as drug-racing) are achievable, but again limited to the relatively few drug-classes with multiple effective medications for HF. Go and colleagues[21] compared the effectiveness of alternative β-blockers in treatment of HF using a pharmacy, clinical, and administrative databases. This clean interclass comparison showed that observational drug-drug CER is extremely beneficial when done properly. Go and colleagues generated important hypotheses and concluded that more trials data would be preferred regarding the interclass effectiveness of β-blockers in HF.

Observational drug-related safety studies can identify, modify, and refine important safety signals that are difficult to detect in most RCTs (which are typically underpowered for adverse drug effects) or not anticipated at the time the RCT was planned or conducted. Drug safety studies require large numbers of patients to investigate the relations between drug use and rare events, which are often unanswered in an effectiveness-driven RCT design. Depending on the adverse event being studied, drug safety analyses may not be as susceptible to treatment selection as in analyses focused on effectiveness of therapies. Because a treatment (eg, β-blockers) is prescribed for a specific reason (eg, systolic HF), it is hard to compare the effectiveness of a β-blocker with patients not being treated with β-blockers, because the indication for receiving this therapy may be directly linked to the outcome of interest (eg, cardiovascular mortality), leading to a biased estimate of the impact of β-blockers on risk of cardiovascular death. However, drug safety studies frequently compare the incidence of an event, which is not an indication or contraindication for treatment or an expected outcome. Hence, if exposure is defined robustly, the comparators are selected logically, and the adverse event is ascertained accurately and comprehensively, the association between exposure and an adverse outcome can be estimated more confidently. Here it is crucial to note that the credibility of large-scale drug safety studies performed on electronic health care data or post hoc analyses from pooled RCT databases is enhanced by other types of data, such as biologic plausibility and the results from other studies using different designs (case studies, epidemiologic reports, trial findings in other settings or similar drugs).

STRENGTHS AND LIMITATIONS OF DRUG-DRUG CER

Optimally, large RCTs would be conducted for every possible treatment option for a target clinical population, and those data would guide therapeutic decision-making for the physician and the patient. Unfortunately, this is not feasible and as noted previously, there are many known limitations of RCTs.[22,23] Therefore, drug-drug CER has an important role in helping to fill important knowledge gaps and can possibly help provide evidence to support future RCTs when results suggest either unforeseen harm or effectiveness of an agent (Fig. 1). However, observational CER studies are inherently limited by the observational nature and only high-quality CER should be included when changing practice guidelines and behaviors. Strengths and limitations are therefore crucial to

realize and must serve as guarantor for the overall responsible reporting of CER. Table 1 lists the overall strengths and limitations of drug-drug CER. Fig. 1 shows the role of CER in the postmarket surveillance of drugs.

Strengths of Drug-Drug CER

The major strength of drug-drug CER is the ability to include a broader study population than traditional RCTs and also to assess the translation of RCT findings into clinical practice. RCTs typically often exclude patients based on selected demographic criteria, comorbidity, disease severity, and concomitant treatments. In addition, patients enrolled in RCTs are often quite different from real world persons who will use the drugs tested in the RCT (eg, elderly, young, unemployed patients, uninsured patients, persons of color). Observational CER can study an entire target population unrelated to geography and therefore add important information regarding safety and effectiveness in patient subgroups not enrolled in RCTs. Observational CER studies are usually able to be completed in a much shorter period of time and with fewer resources compared with RCTs. Another strength of CER is the ability to study large populations efficiently with a high degree of statistical power, although any observed differences between exposure groups need to be evaluated for clinically relevant and not just statistically significant effects. Multiple drug-drug comparisons are also an important advantage of CER because RCTs often only compare a drug with placebo or with one other drug. By rigorously comparing outcomes associated with multiple drugs within a drug class or by comparing classes of drugs, providers could potentially be better informed

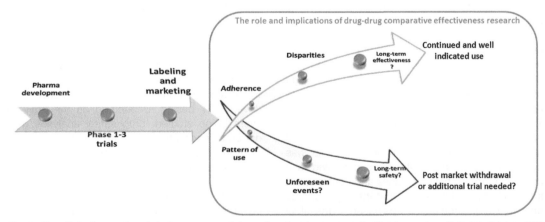

Fig. 1. Simplistic figure showing the process of drug development to marketing to postmarket monitoring. The *blue outlined box* represents the position and role of drug-drug comparative effectiveness research in the field of postmarket drug surveillance.

Table 1
Strengths and limitations of drug-drug comparative effectiveness research

Strengths		Limitations
Real-world clinical practice setting	Drug-drug comparative effectiveness research	Nonrandomized
Broader inclusion of subjects representative of the target population (eg, elderly, young, uninsured patients, all races, and other sociodemographic factors)		No direct information about treatment indication (confounding-by-indication)
Power		Information regarding adherence
Multiple drug-drug comparisons		Treatment selection bias
Ability to study unforeseen effects		Often limited clinical information (blood pressure, biomarkers, and so forth)
Ability to study long-term outcomes		Residual confounding and imperfect risk adjustment
Often more generalizable than trials		Typically less information on disease severity
Faster to conduct		Risk of misinterpretation

regarding the possible benefit of a newer drug versus older drugs. In addition, drug-drug interactions could potentially influence prognosis substantially and especially in the elderly part of the population. Drug-drug interactions and the clinical impact can much more easily be studied using a CER design than by a trial.

Limitations of Drug-Drug CER

Observational CER is inherently limited by the lack of randomization and this introduces the most important limitations of drug-drug CER: treatment selection caused by confounding by indication or confounding by contraindication. We often have no information about the precise reasons why a specific patient received a particular drug. Thus, the disease or the symptom preceding a condition being treated with the drug of interest could alone indicate a condition associated with an increased risk of the studied outcome or death, thus introducing the risk of confounding-by-indication. "Confounding-by-indication" is a commonly used term that refers to an irrelevant determinant of the outcome of interest that is present if a perceived high-risk or poor prognosis is an indication for the therapy.[24] The indication for treatment may be a confounder because it is correlated with receiving the intervention and is a risk indicator for the outcome. Thus, an imbalance in these types of factors between treatment groups can be created based on the chosen exposure. This important bias can be challenging to mitigate using claims data alone and cannot be completely excluded in observational studies. Several design and statistical techniques have been developed to try to reduce the impact of

confounding by indication or confounding by contraindication.

Claims databases often include demographic information and data on comorbidity based on diagnostic and procedural administrative codes but do not include detailed patient or clinical data (eg, individual-level socioeconomic information, lifestyle factor status, weight, vital sign measurements, anthropometry, laboratory test results, pathology results). Systematic differences in adherence to treatment is also a possible bias in studies using pharmacy claims data, which rely on algorithms based on observed refill patterns to estimate longitudinal drug exposure rather than actual documentation of the amount and timing of medication taken by a patient. Nonadherence would typically lead to biasing toward the null because there would be an overestimation of the amount of drug-exposed time and possible misclassification in assigning adverse events to periods of "exposure" when it was not really true.

In summary, drug-drug CER has a variety of important limitations, which should be accounted for in detail in the study design and analytic approaches. Potential biases and confounders should be acknowledged and the interpretation of the results formulated in a cautious, balanced manner to place the CER findings in the proper context.

DRUG-DRUG CER IN HF

Drug-drug CER studies have pointed to a variety of agents that are contraindicated in HF and others have raised concerns about possible safety issues for various drugs in the setting of HF.[25–27] Contrary to this, CER-studies have also examined and strengthened the evidence for effectiveness of selected evidence based medications in HF when used in typical clinical practice settings.[21,28–31] Importantly, however, there still remains important knowledge gaps regarding the short- and long-term effectiveness and safety of various therapies currently used in many patients with HF.[25] Patients with HF are often frail and unforeseen adverse treatment effects of concomitant medications have proved to be important (ie, antithrombotics,[28] non-steroidal anti-inflammatory drugs [NSAIDs],[27] antiarrhythmic drugs,[32] and hypertension agents[33]). To optimize the longitudinal care of patients with HF, it is important to examine commonly used concomitant agents that constitute a possible clinical problem in HF. In addition, understanding the factors that influence adherence and breaks in treatment in real world settings provide an opportunity to potentially improve the delivery of therapies in a way that is closer to the typical adherence seen in RCTs. Various studies have underlined the long-term effectiveness of the evidence-based medications but also suggest individual differences in effectiveness of individual β-blockers, angiotensin II receptor blockers, and angiotensin-converting enzyme inhibitors in real-life HF-settings.[21,29–31,34,35]

CER of β-Blockers in HF: The Importance of Within-Class Comparisons

Go and colleagues[21] examined the real world comparative effectiveness of different oral β-blockers in the Kaiser Permanente Northern California integrated health care delivery system among a large sample of patients with HF and found that shorter-acting metoprolol tartrate was associated with a relative higher death rate compared with atenolol. Overall summary of results is shown in **Table 2**. This study performed an interclass comparison of different β-blockers and cautioned about the interpretation of the results, and suggested that additional RCTs would be needed to confirm or refute the observed findings. This specific study used rigorous methods for best controlling the inherent bias of confounding-by-indication and importantly restrained their study to comparing β-blockers with β-blockers. This is an important approach in drug-drug CER to minimize certain types of treatment selection bias and to avoid unfair comparisons (ie, compare β-blocker users with nonusers and even with users of a different class of drugs). Kramer and colleagues[31] compared evidence-based β-blockers with non–evidence-based β-blockers for effectiveness using inverse probability weighted estimators and found similar results for β-blockers with and without an evidence-based indication for HF. One-year adjusted mortality rates were 28.3% for those receiving no β-blockers, 22.8% for those on non–evidence-based β-blockers, and 24.2% for those on evidence-based β-blockers.

When Drug-Drug CER Creates Dilemmas Regarding Drug Effectiveness: Angiotensin II Receptor Blockers As An Example

A recent study by Eklind-Cervenka and colleagues[29] is an important example of drug-drug CER. In this study, the investigators show a marked difference in risk of mortality associated with two angiotensin II receptor blockers, losartan and candesartan, used in a large HF registry. They

Table 2
Multivariate association between receipt of selected β-blockers and the risk of death within 12 months after discharge[a]

	Compared with Atenolol, Adjusted HR for Death (95% CI)[b]			
	Metoprolol Tartrate	Carvedilol	Other β-Blockers	No β-Blocker
Overall cohort (N = 11326)	1.16 (1.01–1.34)	1.16 (0.92–1.44)	1.04 (0.79–1.37)	1.63 (1.44–1.84)
Subgroup with documented left ventricular systolic dysfunction (N = 2929)	1.14 (0.78–1.67)	1.42 (0.94–2.16)	1.34 (0.68–2.63)	1.85 (1.33–2.57)

Abbreviations: CI, confidence interval; HR, hazard ratio.
  [a] Analyses were conducted in 11,326 adults discharged alive after hospitalization for heart failure between January 1, 2001, and December 31, 2003, and the subgroup of 2379 patients who survived the index hospitalization and who were concurrently receiving digoxin therapy during follow-up. Receipt of digoxin was used as a proxy for the presence of reduced left ventricular systolic function. The reference group was those who received atenolol.
  [b] Models were adjusted for site, calendar year of entry, age, gender, time-varying medical insurance status, baseline propensity score (deciles) for receiving carvedilol, prior hospitalization for heart failure, index hospitalization length of stay, cardiovascular history, other comorbid conditions, and time-varying use of targeted medications.
  From Go AS, Yang J, Gurwitz JH, et al. Comparative effectiveness of different beta-adrenergic antagonists on mortality among adults with heart failure in clinical practice. Arch Intern Med 2008;168:2415–21; with permission.

found that among 30,254 patients with HF, 10% of candesartan users versus 17% of losartan users died at 1 year. At 5-year follow-up, crude mortality risk was also lower among candesartan versus losartan users (39% vs 56%, respectively). In adjusted analysis, losartan was associated with a 43% increased relative risk of death (hazard ratio, 1.43; 95% confidence interval [CI], 1.23–1.65). The implications for this study are clear, but now academic societies are faced with the natural dilemma that drug-drug CER will create: are the findings from this observational study strong enough to recommend a change in practice now or should it be used to push for a new head-to-head RCT? Importantly, however, this finding was not reproduced in a very similar setting,[36] which questions the original report by Eklind-Cervenka. The Eklind-Cervenka study showed a significant relationship with candesartan and death, whereas the Svanstrom study did not. Svanstrom and colleagues[36] found that compared with candesartan, losartan was not associated with increased all-cause mortality (adjusted hazard ratio, 1.10; 95% CI, 0.96–1.25) during follow-up of up to 11 years. The studies were conducted in very similar settings (Sweden and Denmark, respectively). Thus, for this specific example, drug-drug CER did not provide definitive answers, but merely raised more questions. This highlights the importance of evaluating the evidence derived from CER studies of specific drug-drug comparisons and what implications for clinical practice or RCT planning emerge from those studies.

Drug-Drug Comparative Safety Studies in HF

The Acute Study of Clinical Effectiveness of Nesiritide in Decompensated Heart Failure trial (ASCEND-HF) is another recent example of the role of drug-drug CER. ASCEND-HF was initiated after two small meta-analyses had suggested that the recombinantly produced intravenous formulation of human B-type natriuretic peptide, nesiritide, was unsafe in the treatment of acute decompensated HF. The main results of ASCEND-HF showed that nesiritide indeed was safe, but not any more effective than placebo.[37] Readmission for HF or death at 30 days postdischarge was 9.4% in the nesiritide arm versus 10.1% in the placebo arm (*P* = .31). Well-designed drug-drug CER is crucial and ASCEND-HF illustrates that observational studies should be interpreted carefully.

Another recent example of the role of drug-drug safety studies is the evidence building for the class of glucose lowering drugs called thiazolidinediones ("glitazones"). Rosiglitazone was recently withdrawn from the European market after

observational studies had shown that this drug increased the risk of cardiovascular adverse events (including HF) compared with pioglitazone. Graham and colleagues[38] found that HF events were more common in those using rosiglitazone (3.94 events per 100 person-years) versus those using pioglitazone (3 events per 100 person-years), with an adjusted 25% increased relative risk (95% CI, 16%–34%). The corresponding number-needed-to-harm was 106, meaning that for every 106 patients treated with rosiglitazone instead of pioglitazone, one additional HF-related hospitalization would occur. For an overall composite cardiac outcome (myocardial infarction, stroke, HF, or death), the number-needed-to-harm was 60 favoring pioglitazone over rosiglitazone therapy. The European Medicine Agency based their decision of withdrawal mainly on results derived from observational data. Although this may be warranted, it also makes it less likely that a head-to-head RCT comparing all of the different "glitazones" will be performed to more definitively answer the question.

NSAIDs have also been associated with adverse cardiovascular events in HF. NSAIDs are contraindicated for HF because of documented risk of fluid retention properties and the risk of exacerbating HF through pulmonary edema and increasing peripheral edema. Yet, NSAIDs are still used by one in three patients with HF on a national scale representing a substantial public health issue.[27] In a study examining the cardiovascular safety of NSAIDs, Gislason and colleagues[27] found that the risk of rehospitalization for HF and myocardial infarction was substantially increased when associated with use of NSAIDs. In addition, selective cyclooxygenase-2 inhibitors were associated with a higher risk relative to use of traditional NSAIDs or no use of NSAIDs. The results were further underlined by a dose-response relationship and were similar for all-cause mortality (**Fig. 2**). Again, this was an example of a postmarketing assessment of commonly used drugs to delineate an important drug-related risk. Previous RCTs did not perform placebo comparisons or were not powered to examine this relationship, but because of drug-drug safety studies, RCTS are now being conducted to secure the safety of patients with HF in need of NSAID treatment.

Although RCTs are still considered the gold standard for therapeutic decision-making, rigorously conducted drug-drug CER should play an important role in helping to guide the design and conduct of future RCTs, which in turn could help improve translation of research into clinical practice. In addition, many of the methods used in drug-drug CER studies directly apply to

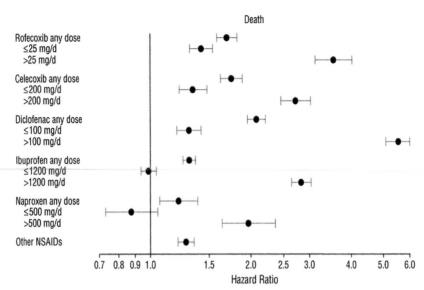

Fig. 2. Hazard ratios for death associated with use of nonsteroidal anti-inflammatory drugs (NSAIDs) in patients with chronic heart failure. Cox proportional hazards regression analysis adjusted for age, gender, calendar year, comorbidity, concomitant pharmacotherapy, and severity of disease. *Bars* indicate 95% confidence intervals. (*From* Gislason GH, Rasmussen JN, Abildstrom SZ, et al. Increased mortality and cardiovascular morbidity associated with use of nonsteroidal anti-inflammatory drugs in chronic heart failure. Arch Intern Med 2009;169:141–9; with permission.)

device-related CER, which is needed given the paucity of adequately powered RCTs comparing devices with each other or devices with other therapeutic strategies. This is becoming particularly relevant in HF because an increasing number of devices have entered the treatment options in HF (eg, implantable cardioverter defibrillator, cardiac resynchronization therapy, left ventricular assist devices). Although there is a long way to prospective automated drug/device surveillance[39] it is undoubtedly a field where CER should expand to improve the robustness of results from postmarket safety and effectiveness studies.

SUMMARY

Drug-drug CER is valuable when applied to the right question using the right methods in a relevant context. Being aware of limitations and strengths, and incorporating these insights into the interpretation of results is crucial. Rigorously performed drug-drug CER can help guide clinical practice and future research in HF.

REFERENCES

1. Tricoci P, Allen JM, Kramer JM, et al. Scientific evidence underlying the ACC/AHA clinical practice guidelines. JAMA 2009;301:831–41.
2. Chalkidou K. From research to health care practice: How the UK uses data on comparative effectiveness. Interview by Bridget M. Kuehn. JAMA 2010;304: 1058–9.
3. Keyhani S, Woodward M, Federman AD. Physician views on the use of comparative effectiveness research: a national survey. Ann Intern Med 2010;153:551–2.
4. Kindig D, Mullahy J. Comparative effectiveness–of what?: evaluating strategies to improve population health. JAMA 2010;304:901–2.
5. Mitka M. US government kicks off program for comparative effectiveness research. JAMA 2010; 304:2230–1.
6. Sox HC. Comparative effectiveness research: a progress report. Ann Intern Med 2010;153:469–72.
7. Schneeweiss S. A basic study design for expedited safety signal evaluation based on electronic healthcare data. Pharmacoepidemiol Drug Saf 2010;19:858–68.
8. Committee on Comparative Effectiveness Research Prioritization, Institute of Medicine. Board on health care services (HCS). Book: initial national priorities for comparative effectiveness research (2009). 2009. Available at: http://www.nap.edu/catalog.php?record_id=12648.
9. Hammill BG, Hernandez AF, Peterson ED, et al. Linking inpatient clinical registry data to Medicare claims data using indirect identifiers. Am Heart J 2009;157: 995–1000.
10. Ray WA. Evaluating medication effects outside of clinical trials: new-user designs. Am J Epidemiol 2003;158:915–20.
11. Schneeweiss S, Avorn J. A review of uses of health care utilization databases for epidemiologic

research on therapeutics. J Clin Epidemiol 2005;58: 323–37.

12. Kelsey J, Whittemore AS, Evans AS, et al. Methods in observational epidemiology. New York: Oxford University Pres; 1996. p. 341–90.

13. Suissa S. Immortal time bias in pharmaco-epidemiology. Am J Epidemiol 2008;167:492–9.

14. Suissa S. Immortal time bias in observational studies of drug effects. Pharmacoepidemiol Drug Saf 2007; 16:241–9.

15. Suissa S. Effectiveness of inhaled corticosteroids in chronic obstructive pulmonary disease: immortal time bias in observational studies. Am J Respir Crit Care Med 2003;168:49–53.

16. Leonardi S, Newby LK, Ohman EM, et al. American Heart Association annual meeting abstract: lack of implementation of ESC/ACC definition of myocardial infarction in contemporary randomized clinical trials. Circulation 2010;122:A11021.

17. Kaul S, Diamond GA. Trial and error. How to avoid commonly encountered limitations of published clinical trials. J Am Coll Cardiol 2010;55:415–27.

18. Kip KE, Hollabaugh K, Marroquin OC, et al. The problem with composite end points in cardiovascular studies: the story of major adverse cardiac events and percutaneous coronary intervention. J Am Coll Cardiol 2008;51:701–7.

19. Alpert JS, Thygesen K. A new global definition of myocardial infarction for the 21st century. Pol Arch Med Wewn 2007;117:485–6.

20. Thygesen K, Alpert JS, White HD, et al. Universal definition of myocardial infarction. Circulation 2007; 116:2634–53.

21. Go AS, Yang J, Gurwitz JH, et al. Comparative effectiveness of different beta-adrenergic antagonists on mortality among adults with heart failure in clinical practice. Arch Intern Med 2008;168:2415–21.

22. Black N. Why we need observational studies to evaluate the effectiveness of health care. BMJ 1996;312:1215–8.

23. Sanson-Fisher RW, Bonevski B, Green LW, et al. Limitations of the randomized controlled trial in evaluating population-based health interventions. Am J Prev Med 2007;33:155–61.

24. Salas M, Hofman A, Stricker BH. Confounding by indication: an example of variation in the use of epidemiologic terminology. Am J Epidemiol 1999;149:981–3.

25. Amabile CM, Spencer AP. Keeping your patient with heart failure safe: a review of potentially dangerous medications. Arch Intern Med 2004;164:709–20.

26. Fosbol EL, Gislason GH, Poulsen HE, et al. Prognosis in heart failure and the value of {beta}-blockers are altered by the use of antidepressants and depend on the type of antidepressants used. Circ Heart Fail 2009;2:582–90.

27. Gislason GH, Rasmussen JN, Abildstrom SZ, et al. Increased mortality and cardiovascular morbidity associated with use of nonsteroidal anti-inflammatory drugs in chronic heart failure. Arch Intern Med 2009;169:141–9.

28. Bonde L, Sorensen R, Fosbol EL, et al. Increased mortality associated with low use of clopidogrel in patients with heart failure and acute myocardial infarction not undergoing percutaneous coronary intervention: a nationwide study. J Am Coll Cardiol 2010;55:1300–7.

29. Eklind-Cervenka M, Benson L, Dahlstrom U, et al. Association of candesartan vs losartan with all-cause mortality in patients with heart failure. JAMA 2011;305:175–82.

30. Hernandez AF, Hammill BG, O'Connor CM, et al. Clinical effectiveness of beta-blockers in heart failure: findings from the optimize-HF (organized program to initiate lifesaving treatment in hospitalized patients with heart failure) registry. J Am Coll Cardiol 2009;53:184–92.

31. Kramer JM, Curtis LH, Dupree CS, et al. Comparative effectiveness of beta-blockers in elderly patients with heart failure. Arch Intern Med 2008;168:2422–8 [discussion: 2428–32].

32. Echt DS, Liebson PR, Mitchell LB, et al. Mortality and morbidity in patients receiving encainide, flecainide, or placebo. The cardiac Arrhythmia Suppression Trial. N Engl J Med 1991;324:781–8.

33. Yusuf S, Sleight P, Pogue J, et al. Effects of an angiotensin-converting-enzyme inhibitor, ramipril, on cardiovascular events in high-risk patients. The Heart Outcomes Prevention Evaluation Study investigators. N Engl J Med 2000;342:145–53.

34. Allen LaPointe NM, Zhou Y, Stafford JA, et al. Association between mortality and persistent use of beta blockers and angiotensin-converting enzyme inhibitors in patients with left ventricular systolic dysfunction and coronary artery disease. Am J Cardiol 2009; 103:1518–24.

35. Gislason GH, Rasmussen JN, Abildstrom SZ, et al. Persistent use of evidence-based pharmacotherapy in heart failure is associated with improved outcomes. Circulation 2007;116:737–44.

36. Svanstrom H, Pasternak B, Hviid A. Association of treatment with losartan vs candesartan and mortality among patients with heart failure. JAMA 2012;307: 1506–12.

37. O'Connor CM, Starling RC, Hernandez AF, et al. Effect of nesiritide in patients with acute decompensated heart failure. [Erratum in: N Engl J Med. 2011;365(8):773.] Wilson, W H [corrected to Tang, W H W]. N Engl J Med 2011;365(1):32–43.

38. Graham DJ, Ouellet-Hellstrom R, MaCurdy TE, et al. Risk of acute myocardial infarction, stroke, heart failure, and death in elderly Medicare patients treated with rosiglitazone or pioglitazone. JAMA 2010;304:411–8.

39. Rumsfeld JS, Peterson ED. Achieving meaningful device surveillance: from reaction to proaction. JAMA 2010;304:2065–6.

Heart Failure Patient Adherence
Epidemiology, Cause, and Treatment

Paul S. Corotto, MD[a], Melissa M. McCarey, BA[b],
Suzanne Adams, RN, MPH[b], Prateeti Khazanie, MD, MPH[c],
David J. Whellan, MD, MHS[b],*

KEYWORDS

- Heart failure • Adherence • Compliance • Self management

KEY POINTS

- Poor adherence to therapeutic regimens is a significant impediment to improving clinical outcomes in the heart failure (HF) population.
- Typical rates of adherence to prescribed medications, low-sodium diets, and aerobic exercise programs remain lower than those needed to decrease morbidity and mortality associated with HF.
- Factors contributing to poor adherence include multiple comorbidities, clinical depression, decreased cognitive functioning, and medication costs.
- HF education and programs to enhance self-management skills have improved patient quality of life but have yet to decrease mortality or rehospitalization rates significantly.
- Telemonitoring to improve adherence behaviors and self-management interventions within broader HF management programs have demonstrated significant clinical improvements in this population.

The American Heart Association (AHA) has identified adherence as an integral component in HF self-care.[1] Unfortunately, adherence to medication, diet, and exercise regimens historically has been poor. This review discusses relevant literature related to poor adherence in several therapeutic domains, including the factors contributing to poor adherence, interventions designed to improve adherence, and HF self-management programs.

ADHERENCE
Defining Medication Adherence

Medication adherence has been classically defined by the percentage of prescribed doses taken over a specific period of time. Patients are typically described as adherent when they take greater than or equal to 80% of their prescribed medications. This parameter is arbitrary and does not account for those who take more than the prescribed amount.[2] In their 2005 review of medication adherence, Osterberg and Blaschke[2] noted that the evaluation of adherence itself can be problematic. Direct methods of observation, such as the measured concentration of a drug or a metabolite, are often limited by both financial and time constraints. In contrast, indirect methods, such as patient questionnaires, medication diaries, rates of prescription refills, and pill counts, can result in the overestimation of patient

Funding support: N/A.
The authors have nothing to disclose.
[a] UPMC Internal Medicine, UPMC Montefiore Hospital, University of Pittsburgh Medical Center, 200 Lothrop Street, N-713, Pittsburgh, PA 15213, USA; [b] Coordinating Center for Clinical Research, Department of Medicine, Jefferson Medical College, 1015 Chestnut Street, Suite 317, Philadelphia, PA 19107, USA; [c] Division of Cardiology, Duke University, Suite 7400, 40 Duke Medicine Circle, Durham, NC 27705, USA
* Corresponding author.
E-mail address: david.whellan@jefferson.edu

Heart Failure Clin 9 (2013) 49–58
http://dx.doi.org/10.1016/j.hfc.2012.09.004
1551-7136/13/$ – see front matter © 2013 Elsevier Inc. All rights reserved.

adherence. Even the common use of pill counts as a simple method to assess adherence has been questioned.[3,4]

Adherence and Mortality

There is some evidence that medication adherence may provide benefits beyond the therapeutic benefit of the medication itself. In particular, several clinical trials have demonstrated that medication adherence has a negative association with mortality. The Coronary Drug Project[5] was one of the first studies to demonstrate this phenomenon. This analysis looked at 1103 men treated with clofibrate and 2789 men given placebo. The study showed that in the treatment arm, 5-year mortality for good adherers (patients who took greater than or equal to 80% of study medication) was 15% compared with 24.6% for poor adherers (P = .00011). The placebo group, however, showed similar results with 5-year mortality at 15.1% for good adherers and 28.3% for poor adherers (P = 4.7×10^{-16}). The Beta-Blocker Heart Attack Trial[6] also demonstrated the effect of adherence on mortality. This study compared the β-blocker propanalol with placebo in patients who had experienced an acute myocardial infarction. Overall, patients who did not adhere to their treatment (took less than 75% of their medication) had higher 1-year mortality rates than patients who did were adherent (odds ratio [OR] 2.6). This effect was observed in both the treatment group (OR 3.1) and the placebo group (OR 2.5).

Medication Adherence

The literature has shown that adherence to HF medications is particularly poor. A 2008 meta-analysis by Wu and colleagues[7] found medication nonadherence rates in HF patients to range typically from 40% to 60%, with some studies reporting values as extreme as 10% to 92%. This range of nonadherence was consistent across multiple methods of measurement, including self-report, pharmacy refill data, medication event monitoring systems, and pill counts. Other studies have also illustrated straightforward yet substantial barriers to medication adherence. Less than 40% of HF patients seen in emergency departments could read their medication label or state the prescribed dose or frequency. The same study found that less than 15% of the patients could properly describe the indication of each medication.[8] In a 2004 study by Butler and colleagues,[9] the investigators followed 960 patients with HF and found that only 77% of the patients filled their prescription for an angiotensin-converting enzyme inhibitor (ACEI)

within 30 days and that more than 63% were using the medication 1 year after discharge.

Poor adherence to HF medications has been repeatedly demonstrated to bear substantial clinical significance. In a study aimed at determining an objective level of medication adherence associated with improved clinical outcomes, Wu and colleagues[10] measured medication adherence in 135 HF patients over a 3.5-year period. The study used the Medication Event Monitoring System (MEMS), a microelectronic monitoring device in the caps of medication vials that records the date and time that the cap is removed. The MEMS allowed the investigators to track both the percentage of prescribed doses taken and the percentage of days that the correct number of doses was taken. The investigators found that an adherence rate of 88% or more to the most common HF medications (β-blockers, ACEI diuretics, and digoxin) was associated with a significantly improved event-free survival rate.

Larger studies of medication adherence in HF patients have also demonstrated survival advantages when evaluating specific therapeutic agents. The Organized Program to Initiate Life-saving Treatment in Hospitalized Patients with Heart Failure (OPTIMIZE-HF) used β-blocker drugs in HF patients with left-ventricular systolic dysfunction to determine if this class of drug offers an early survival benefit to patients postdischarge. More than 1100 patients were prescribed the medication at the time of hospital discharge and were then evaluated between 60 days and 90 days postdischarge. The use of a β-blocker was associated with a significant reduction in the adjusted risk of death (hazard ratio [HR] 0.48; 95% CI, 0.32–0.74; P<.001) and death/rehospitalization (OR 0.74; 95% CI, 0.55–0.99; P = .04).[11] Of note, 93.1% of the participants were found adhering to their prescribed medical regimen during this 60-day to 90-day interval. These data coupled with that described by Wu and colleagues illustrates the substantial gap between the ideal levels of adherence required to improve clinical outcomes and those currently achieved by the HF population.

Dietary Adherence

The ability of patients to follow a low-sodium diet has also been analyzed in relation to treatment adherence in HF. One of greatest obstacles to addressing the issue of dietary adherence has been the lack of consistency in published guidelines regarding recommended sodium intake in the HF population. For example, the Heart Failure Society of America practice guidelines released in 2010 suggest an intake of 2 g to 3 g of sodium per day[5] whereas the American College of Cardiology and the AHA (ACC/AHA) 2005 guidelines recommend between 3 g and 4 g per day.[12] This inconsistency in published recommendations of daily sodium intake for patients with HF represents a lack of controlled trials investigating this parameter.[1]

Although the recommended sodium intake for HF patients remains ambiguous, current literature shows that many HF patients have a daily intake exceeding any published recommendations. Data obtained from the National Health and Nutrition Examination Surveys (NHANES) from 1999 through 2006 showed that 32% of HF patients have a daily sodium intake greater than 3 g and that 15% exceed 4 g daily.[13] The difficulty of adhering to dietary recommendations is further compounded by many HF patients denying any knowledge that such recommendations exist.

A study by Lainscak and colleagues[14] examined data obtained from more than 2300 HF patients 12 weeks after discharge from the hospital. They determined that approximately 40% of patients did not recall receiving advice regarding sodium intake. Of those patients who did recall such advice, only 40% reported to have actually followed the advice.

In a study of patients referred to a specialty clinic for assessment, only 14% were aware of sodium restriction guidelines at a baseline assessment and only 58% were able to read the sodium content from a standard nutrition facts label.[15] Therefore, dietary adherence in the HF population seems to suffer from both a lack of consistency in recommended guidelines as well as an inherent deficiency in relaying the significance of dietary restrictions to the patients themselves.

Exercise Adherence

Although not as thoroughly studied over time as medication and dietary interventions, routine physical activity has become an accepted aspect of HF treatment regimens in recent years and is part of the Heart Failure Society of America and AHA/ACC guidelines. In their 2003 statement on exercise and heart railure, the AHA cites several clinical trials demonstrating the positive effects of exercise, including improved ventilatory response, heart rate variability, peak cardiac index, and indices of diastolic function.[16] Beyond these improvements in physiologic parameters, studies have also shown clinical benefits to exercise regimens in HF patients.

Belardinelli and colleagues[17] randomized 99 patients with documented stable HF to either a standardized exercise regimen group or a control group. This study demonstrated both a higher mortality rate for patients in the control group (relative risk [RR] 0.37, $P = .01$) and a lower hospital readmission rate for HF in the group that completed the exercise regimen (RR 0.29, $P = .02$).

The Exercise Rehabilitation Trial[18] examined the effects of exercise training on 6-minute walk performance, peak oxygen uptake, and arm and leg strength. One hundred eighty-one patients with HF were randomized the exercise training group or the usual care group. The exercise training group received 3 months of supervised exercise training followed by 9 months of home-based exercise training. Both groups displayed significant increases in 6-minute walk duration at 3 and 12 months. The exercise group showed incremental peak oxygen uptake at 3 and 12 months compared with the control group. The exercise group also showed significant increases for arm and leg strength compared with the control group. Patients in the treatment group had high rates of adherence to the supervised exercise sessions; however, adherence declined during the home-based sessions. During the first month of home-based training, patients participated in an average of 2.3 sessions per week and 1.7 sessions per week during the twelfth month.[18]

The Heart Failure: A Controlled Trial Investigating Outcomes of Exercise Training (HF-ACTION) trial was a larger and more comprehensive investigation of the effects of a standardized exercise regimen in this population.[19] This study was a multicenter trial that randomized 2331 patients with stable HF and a left ventricular ejection fraction greater than or equal to 35 to either exercise training or usual care. The aerobic exercise regimen was found to decrease all-cause mortality or all-cause hospitalization, the primary endpoint (HR 0.93 [95% CI, 0.84–1.02]; $P = .13$; HR, after adjusting for highly predictive baseline characteristics, 0.89 [95% CI, 0.81–0.99]; $P = .03$). It also demonstrated significant improvement in subject reported quality of life at the 3-month interval.

Despite significant effort to maintain adherence to the exercise regimen evaluated in HF-ACTION, the participants within the exercise group had difficulty maintaining to the training schedule. Those in the intervention group exercised for a median of 76 minutes per week (interquartile range, 39–117 minutes per week). The exercise training goal during this time was 90 minutes per week, with the exercise time increased to a median of 95 minutes per week (interquartile range, 26–184 minutes per week) at 4 to 6 months after enrollment. They subsequently decreased to a median of 74 minutes per week (interquartile range, 0–180 minutes per week) at 10 to 12 months after enrollment, with a training goal of

120 minutes per week. In the third year of follow-up, patients in the exercise training group were exercising a median of 50 minutes per week (interquartile range, 0–140 minutes per week). At all time points, only 30% or more of the patients in the exercise training group exercised at or above the target exercise minutes per week. The drop-off in exercise adherence was similar to the study performed by McKelvie and colleagues.

These data in HF-ACTION supports previous studies that demonstrated HF patients as poor at engaging in regular exercise routines. In a study of 139 HF patients with an average age of just above 69 years, Carlson and colleagues[20] found that more than 53% of the participants reported engaging in no physical activity each week. A needs-assessment survey conducted by Ni and colleagues[21] found that 35% of those assessed were active fewer than twice per month. Although exercise regimens are currently recommended by the AHA/ACC as an adjunctive treatment in patients with HF, the poor adherence rates along with the historically low rates of physical activity in this population illustrates the significant difficulty in implementing such programs into routine HF therapy.

FACTORS AFFECTING ADHERENCE
Comorbid Conditions

Adherence to a treatment regimen is often impaired by factors inherent to HF, in particular the multiple comorbidities that often affect HF patients. The Acute Decompensated Heart Failure National Registry of more than 60,000 patients with HF showed that 56% had coronary artery disease, more than 70% had hypertension, more than 30% had hyperlipidemia, and more than 40% had diabetes.[22] This high prevalence of comorbid conditions has a substantial impact on both medication and dietary adherence in patients with HF.[23] Multiple comorbidities affect medication adherence in several distinct ways; the most basic involves the sheer number of medications required to treat these conditions.[24,25] Martinez-Selles and colleagues[25] found that 74% of HF subjects evaluated were taking 6 or more medications.

The high number of medications can lead to confusion regarding the reason a patient is taking a medication. In the same study by Martinez-Selles and colleagues,[25] only half of patients taking β-blockers knew that the medication decreased blood pressure, fewer than 40% recognized the action of spironolactone, and more than 10% did not know that diuretics help to eliminate liquids from the body. The presence of multiple comorbidities also results in greater difficulties in symptom monitoring. For instance, a patient suffering from both HF and chronic lung disease may have difficulty interpreting the source of the dyspnea and thus may fail to increase the dose of a diuretic during a HF exacerbation. To further compound this issue, it has been shown that as the number of comorbid conditions increases, so does the likelihood of the patient to attribute their symptoms to age-related changes.[26]

Depression

It has been long been understood that patients suffering from a chronic disease are prone to developing significant mood disturbances, including clinical depression. In this light, several studies have demonstrated the significant prevalence of depression in the HF population. Jiang and colleagues found that 35% of 374 hospitalized HF patients screened positive for clinical depression using the Beck Depression Inventory.[27] Likewise, Gottlieb and colleagues[28] demonstrated that the rate of clinical depression was 48% in 155 ambulatory patients with HF, a rate much higher than that of the general population.

Clinical depression in HF patients can adversely affects adherence to treatment regimens. Morgan and colleagues[29] questioned whether patient-reported difficulties in taking medications could be explained by the concurrent presence of depression. In their study, 44% of patients who reported having difficulty taking medications as prescribed had depressive symptoms compared with only 37% of those who did not report such difficulties ($P = .006$).[29]

The role of depression in reducing adherence rates has also been shown in other forms of heart disease. Gehi and colleagues[30] found that depressed patients with coronary disease were twice as likely to report forgetting to take their medications as nondepressed patients. Furthermore, depressed patients were more than twice as likely to admit to skip their medications purposefully. These trends persisted even when confounding variables, such as age, ethnicity, and education level, were properly controlled.

Current literature lacks data supporting a causative relationship between depression and decreased adherence in HF. The well-documented prevalence of depression in this population, however, in conjunction with data supporting a causative relationship in other forms of heart disease suggests that improved treatment of depression in HF patients may improve adherence.

Impaired Cognition

Up to 17% of people over the age of 65 years demonstrate at least mildly diminished cognitive function,[31] and there is an even higher prevalence of impaired cognition in HF patients than in the population at large.[32,33] There is also evidence to support the notion that decreased cognitive ability is directly associated with poor HF self-care practices.[34] Therefore, a greater understanding of the relationship between HF and cognitive impairment is vital when considering factors that lead to decreased therapeutic adherence.

Two major mechanisms proposed to explain the pathophysiology of impaired cognition in the setting of HF are cardioembolic events and reduced perfusion. Neuroimaging studies of HF patients support both mechanisms, demonstrating significant evidence of gray matter damage in cortical regions key to cognitive functioning as well as a decline in cerebral perfusion.[35,36] Left ventricular dysfunction results in increased end-diastolic volume and stasis, a predisposing condition for thrombus formation.[37] Multiple studies have demonstrated that decreased ejection fraction is the strongest risk factor for both ventricular thrombus formation[38] and cerebral infarction.[39] The recurrence of cardioembolic events leading to repeated lacunar strokes results in subsequent dementia. This serves as a possible mechanism to explain the prevalence of cognitive impairment in the HF population.

The second proposed mechanism involves decreased cerebral perfusion.[37] Over time, decreased left ventricular systolic function and subsequent decrease in ejection fraction causes diminished blood flow in both the carotid and vertebrobasilar systems. HF patients have demonstrated reduced cerebrovascular reactivity.[40] They are also unable to maintain normal cerebral perfusion with this reduced cardiac output thus leading to cognitive impairment.

Medication Costs

Another factor that contributes to poor adherence is medication cost. A 2004 study by Piette and colleagues[41] found that 18% of chronically ill patients surveyed reported cutting back on medication use due to cost in the previous year. A diagnosis of HF is usually accompanied by a costly and complex medication regimen. HF patients are commonly on β-blockers, ACEIs, and diuretics as well as a variety of other medications to treat symptoms and comorbid conditions. This complex regimen translates into high medication costs and copays for people with HF. Several investigators have demonstrated associations between high medications costs and poor adherence.

A retrospective cohort study by Patterson and colleagues[42] looked at associations between β-blocker copay cost and β-blocker adherence. The investigators used data from a claims database to determine monthly copay costs and refill frequency for 2359 HF patients over 50 years old. Adherence was determined by medication possession ratio, which is based on the number of calendar days that elapsed between 2 refills. The study showed that patients who were prescribed β-blockers that with copays greater than $20 per month had a 9% annual decrease in yearly β-blocker supply compared with patients who were prescribed β-blockers with monthly copays, which fall between $0 and $5. Another analysis by Dunlay and colleagues[43] looked at medication adherence behaviors among people living in a small community. The patients with poor adherence reported financial difficulties as a barrier to medication adherence. For example, behaviors, such as skipping doses to save money and delaying prescription refills due to cost, were reported more often by patients with poor adherence than patients with good adherence (46% vs 6%; $P<.001$).

INTERVENTIONS TO IMPROVE ADHERENCE

Several forms of intervention designed to enhance adherence to therapeutic regimens within the framework of improved self-management have been studied in recent years (**Table 1**). The literature has concentrated on interventional techniques to enhance HF knowledge and skill development with the broader goal of improving self-management behaviors to subsequently improve clinical outcomes.

The most recent AHA scientific statement on self-care in HF noted that patients must develop the ability to recognize signs and symptoms of the disease. In addition, patients must develop the skills needed to properly implement a change in management of their care.[1] Several studies are discussed that have specifically evaluated the effect of educational intervention on self-care behaviors.

Jaarsma and colleagues[44] studied patients hospitalized with an exacerbation of HF to determine the benefits of formal teaching sessions on topics ranging from signs and symptoms of decompensation to fluid balance and sodium restriction. Patients in the intervention group received an average of 4 inpatient sessions followed by a telephone session within a week of discharge and a subsequent home visit by a nurse. Self-care behavior was assessed by a 19-item questionnaire requiring yes or no answers concerning specific behaviors, such as measuring daily weights. Quality of life was assessed using

Table 1
Studies of interventions to enhance adherence to therapeutic regimens

Study	Intervention	Endpoint	Result
Jaarsma et al,[44] 2000	Self-management teaching sessions	Self-care behaviors and quality of life	Improved self-care behaviors for treatment group. No difference in quality-of-life measures between groups
Harrison et al,[45] 2002	Hospital to home transitional care plan	Readmission rates and emergency department visits	12-Week readmission rate: Treatment group 23% Usual care group 31% Emergency department visits: Treatment group 29% Usual care group 43%
Wright et al,[46] 2003	Self-management program	Knowledge of self-management readmission and mortality	Treatment group displayed better knowledge derived from a composite endpoint of self-management skills measurement. No difference between groups in readmission or mortality rates
Prasun et al,[47] 2005	Diuretic titration education protocol	Exercise ED visits Tolerance Quality-of-life Hospitalizations Mortality	Treatment group displayed increased exercise tolerance and quality of life scores and fewer emergency department visits than treatment group. No difference between groups in hospitalization and mortality
HART	Self-management education		Low socioeconomic status and self-management
WHARF trial	Telemonitoring	Mortality	56% Mortality reduction
Hershberger et al,[50] 2001	Self-management program		52% Reduction in cardiovascular hospitalizations 72%

a multiple-dimensional analysis of functional capabilities, symptoms, and psychosocial perceptions. The investigators found that the structured educational intervention significantly improved self-care behaviors but did not increase quality of life.

Further studies have investigated the inclusion of formal patient education intervention within a broader program aimed at improving the transition from hospitalization to home. In a 12-week randomized trial, Harrison and colleagues[45] compared HF patients treated with usual postdischarge care with patients assigned to a transitional care plan, which consisted of an education booklet, postdischarge home visits by a nurse, and a formal education program using a patient workbook. The workbook included instructions for proper management of diet, medications, and exercise. The transitional care group also had access to a nursing transfer letter that documented their clinical status and self-management needs as well as telephone outreach from a study nurse within 1 day of discharge. The investigators found that the transitional care group demonstrated a significant improvement in quality of life and visited the emergency department less often for HF exacerbations. Harrison and colleagues demonstrated that a focused intervention aimed at increasing a patient's ability to self-manage can have a significant clinical impact in the HF population.

Education and self-management interventions may increase self-care behaviors and quality of life, but it is also necessary to determine if these interventions lead to improved clinical outcomes.

Wright and colleagues[46] randomized patients hospitalized for HF exacerbations into either a management or a usual care group. Participants in the management group were scheduled for an outpatient clinical review within 2 weeks of discharge and then at 6-week intervals for the duration of the 12-month study. Each clinical review included personal counseling and HF education performed by a HF nurse. Medication adjustments were made by a physician. Patients in the management group were also provided with diaries that include contact information for the clinic, a medication list, and a calendar for the recording of daily weights. The patients were instructed to purchase home weight scales if they did not own one and to make predetermined alterations to their management plans if they noted weight changes greater than 2 pounds. They were also encouraged to attend 3 education sessions that emphasized daily weight monitoring, plans of action in the event of weight changes, effects of medications, and suggestions for diet and exercise. The investigators assessed patient knowledge regarding self-management strategies 12 months after discharge for patients in the management and usual care groups as well as primary end points of death and rehospitalization.

The study found that patients in the management group demonstrated greater knowledge of self-management strategies and were also more likely to use those strategies including monitoring of daily weight. The investigators also found that patients in the management group who did not use their weight diaries had a higher rate of missed clinic appointments, a higher mortality rate, and a 50% shorter time to readmission.[46] The study failed to demonstrate, however, a significant difference in mortality or rehospitalization between treatment groups. In all, acquisition of self-management behaviors through educational interventions resulted in a significant positive clinical impact but did not demonstrate a difference in primary outcomes.

Further studies have been conducted to determine if specific aspects of self-management interventions have a significant impact, for example, diuretic titration. A diuretic that can be titrated in response to the patient's changing fluid status serves as a key aspect of most HF therapeutic regimens. Although many patients rely on their physician to titrate the dose of diuretic based on fluid status evaluation in the office, other patients are permitted to self-titrate the dose according to a weight-based protocol.

Prasun and colleagues[47] randomized HF patients into a usual care group or a group using a patient-directed flexible diuretic protocol to determine the effect on clinical outcomes as well as quality of life. The patients in each group were provided with the same education protocol, including information on symptom recognition, diet and exercise recommendations, medication compliance, and self-management strategies that included a scale and diary to record daily weights. Participants in both groups were also given diuretic titration self-assessment questions to be answered daily, but only participants in the experimental group were instructed on how to use the titration protocol to self-adjust their diuretic dose. The study failed to demonstrate a decrease in mortality or rehospitalization for the group instructed on how to self-titrate, but it did demonstrate enhanced quality of life measures and exercise tolerance in the self-titration group.[47] Although each group was provided with the same education regarding standard self-management, the study demonstrated that additional instruction on the management of a specific subset of symptoms can be beneficial.

The randomized trials (discussed previously) have contributed to a better understanding of the utility of self-management interventions in the HF population. Each of the trials, however, failed to demonstrate a significant decrease in either mortality or rehospitalization rates. Powell noted that small sample sizes, low number of intervention sessions, and short durations of evaluation might have contributed to this lack of evidence.[48]

In light of these limitations, the Heart Failure Adherence and Retention Trial (HART) was conducted to determine the benefit of self-management counseling when coupled with standard HF education. Participants randomized into the self-management group took part in 18 2-hour group meetings over the course of a year. The meetings provided educational tip sheets on self-management topics, including medication adherence, sodium restriction, and moderate physical activity. Patients in the intervention group also completed problem-solving challenges designed to develop their self-management skills to properly use the knowledge gained during education sessions. Participants in the control group received the same educational HF tip sheets in the mail at the same time intervals as the intervention group but did not attend in-person meetings. The HART did not find a significant effect of self-management on mortality or rehospitalization; the study demonstrated a significant relationship between self-management and low socioeconomic status, however, and thus opened the door for future studies to investigate this possible relationship.[43]

Other investigators have attempted to determine whether strict adherence to a particular self-management behavior results in improved clinical outcomes. The Weight Monitoring in Heart Failure (WHARF) trial used a telemonitoring system to maintain ideal adherence to daily weighing protocols over a 6-month period. Study participants randomized to the standard care group (N = 142) were instructed to weigh themselves twice daily and to bring these recorded weights to follow-up appointments with their physician.

Participants in the intervention group (N = 138) were instructed to weigh themselves twice daily and to answer a series of yes or no questions pertaining to HF-related symptoms. Study nurses reviewed the data from the intervention group on a daily basis and telephoned patients if significant changes were noted. Compliance with the daily telemonitoring protocol in the intervention group was excellent (98.5% over 6 months), and there was a 56% reduction in mortality in patients randomized to the telemonitoring group (18.4% vs 8%, P<.003). Thus, the WHARF trial illustrated the significance of strict adherence to self-management behaviors in improving clinical outcomes and the potential of telemonitoring systems to vastly improve that adherence.[49]

Other studies have also investigated the role of disease management programs in the improvement of self-care behaviors and therapeutic adherence. Hershberger and colleagues[50] studied the effects of a comprehensive HF management program on both self-care adherence behaviors and clinical outcomes over a 6-month period. Participants in the study were randomized into a control group who received standard of care for HF and an intervention group who received standard of care along with enrollment in the comprehensive program. The program included telemanagement of patients, preemptive hospitalization for decompensating patients, continuity of care from the inpatient to the outpatient setting, and a formal educational program. This formal education included instruction on sodium restriction, pharmacologic therapy, signs and symptoms of decompensation, and behavioral techniques for improving dietary and medication adherence. The self-management and adherence behavior of each participant was ascertained via a needs-assessment survey that was completed at baseline and then again at 6 months. The investigators found significant increases in patient knowledge for participants in the intervention group from baseline to 6 months. The proportion of patients who recognized the importance of daily weight monitoring increased from 53% at baseline to 73% at 6 months (P = .001) and a greater proportion of patients perceived the importance of dietary salt intake restriction (75% vs 83%; P = .01). The study also demonstrated an increase in adherence behaviors in participants within the intervention group; the proportion of patients who weighed themselves daily increased from 43% to 53% (P = .02). Compared with 6 months before referral, the program intervention resulted in a 52% reduction in hospitalizations for cardiovascular causes (56.1% vs 27.2%, P = 001) and a 72% reduction in emergency room visits (53.6% vs 14.5%, P = .01). The work of Hersherberger

and colleagues illustrates the significant improvements in patient adherence and self-management behavior that can be achieved through comprehensive HF management programs. Coupled with the broader improvement in clinical outcomes contributed to this HF management program it demonstrates the significant utility of such programs in HF therapy.

SUMMARY

Poor adherence to therapeutic regimens is a significant impediment to improving clinical outcomes in the HF population. Typical rates of adherence to prescribed medications, low-sodium diets, and aerobic exercise programs remain lower than that needed to decrease morbidity and mortality associated with HF. Factors contributing to poor adherence include multiple comorbidities, clinical depression, and decreased cognitive functioning.

HF education and programs to enhance self-management skills have improved patient quality of life but have yet to decrease mortality or rehospitalization rates significantly. Telemonitoring to improve adherence behaviors and self-management interventions within broader HF management programs have demonstrated significant clinical improvements in this population.

REFERENCES

1. Riegel B, Moser DK, Anker SD, et al. State of the science: promoting self-care in persons with heart failure: a scientific statement from the American Heart Association. Circulation 2009;120:1141–63.
2. Osterberg L, Blaschke T. Adherence to medication. N Engl J Med 2005;353:487–97.
3. Pullar T, Kumar S, Tindall H, et al. Time to stop counting the tablets? Clin Pharmacol Ther 1989;46:163–8.
4. Rudd P, Byyny RL, Zachary V, et al. Pill count measures of compliance in a drug trial: variability and suitability. Am J Hypertens 1988;1:309–12.
5. Heart Failure Society of America. Executive summary: HFSA 2010 Comprehensive Heart Failure Practice Guideline. J Card Fail 2010;16:475–539.
6. Horwitz RI, Viscoli CM, Berkman L, et al. Treatment adherence and risk of death after a myocardial infarction. Lancet 1990;336:542–5.
7. Wu JR, Moser DK, Lennie TA, et al. Medication adherence in patients who have heart failure: a review of the literature. Nurs Clin North Am 2008; 43:133–53, vii–viii.
8. Hope CJ, Wu J, Tu W, et al. Association of medication adherence, knowledge, and skills with emergency department visits by adults 50 years or older with congestive heart failure. Am J Health Syst Pharm 2004;61:2043–9.

9. Butler J, Arbogast PG, Daugherty J, et al. Outpatient utilization of angiotensin-converting enzyme inhibitors among heart failure patients after hospital discharge. J Am Coll Cardiol 2004;43: 2036–43.

10. Wu JR, Moser DK, De Jong MJ, et al. Defining an evidence-based cutpoint for medication adherence in heart failure. Am Heart J 2009;157:285–91.

11. Fonarow GC, Abraham WT, Albert NM, et al. Prospective evaluation of beta-blocker use at the time of hospital discharge as a heart failure performance measure: results from OPTIMIZE-HF. J Card Fail 2007;13:722–31.

12. Hunt SA. ACC/AHA 2005 guideline update for the diagnosis and management of chronic heart failure in the adult: a report of the American College of Cardiology/American Heart Association Task Force on Practice Guidelines (Writing Committee to Update the 2001 Guidelines for the Evaluation and Management of Heart Failure). J Am Coll Cardiol 2005;46:e1–82.

13. Lemon SC, Olendzki B, Magner R, et al. The dietary quality of persons with heart failure in NHANES 1999-2006. J Gen Intern Med 2010;25:135–40.

14. Lainscak M, Cleland JG, Lenzen MJ, et al. Nonpharmacologic measures and drug compliance in patients with heart failure: data from the EuroHeart Failure Survey. Am J Cardiol 2007;99:31D–7D.

15. Neily JB, Toto KH, Gardner EB, et al. Potential contributing factors to noncompliance with dietary sodium restriction in patients with heart failure. Am Heart J 2002;143:29–33.

16. Pina IL, Apstein CS, Balady GJ, et al. Exercise and heart failure: a statement from the American Heart Association Committee on exercise, rehabilitation, and prevention. Circulation 2003;107:1210–25.

17. Belardinelli R, Georgiou D, Cianci G, et al. Randomized, controlled trial of long-term moderate exercise training in chronic heart failure: effects on functional capacity, quality of life, and clinical outcome. Circulation 1999;99:1173–82.

18. McKelvie RS, Teo KK, Roberts R, et al. Effects of exercise training in patients with heart failure: the Exercise Rehabilitation Trial (EXERT). Am Heart J 2002;144:23–30.

19. O'Connor CM, Whellan DJ, Lee KL, et al. Efficacy and safety of exercise training in patients with chronic heart failure: HF-ACTION randomized controlled trial. JAMA 2009;301:1439–50.

20. Carlson B, Riegel B, Moser DK. Self-care abilities of patients with heart failure. Heart Lung 2001;30:351–9.

21. Ni H, Nauman D, Burgess D, et al. Factors influencing knowledge of and adherence to self-care among patients with heart failure. Arch Intern Med 1999;159:1613–9.

22. Fonarow GC, Yancy CW, Heywood JT. Adherence to heart failure quality-of-care indicators in US hospitals: analysis of the ADHERE Registry. Arch Intern Med 2005;165:1469–77.

23. Riegel B, Moser DK, Powell M, et al. Nonpharmacologic care by heart failure experts. J Card Fail 2006; 12:149–53.

24. Lien CT, Gillespie ND, Struthers AD, et al. Heart failure in frail elderly patients: diagnostic difficulties, co-morbidities, polypharmacy and treatment dilemmas. Eur J Heart Fail 2002;4:91–8.

25. Martinez-Selles M, Garcia Robles JA, Munoz R, et al. Pharmacological treatment in patients with heart failure: patients knowledge and occurrence of polypharmacy, alternative medicine and immunizations. Eur J Heart Fail 2004;6:219–26.

26. Rich MW. Heart failure in the elderly: strategies to optimize outpatient control and reduce hospitalizations. Am J Geriatr Cardiol 2003;12:19–24 [quiz: 25–7].

27. Jiang W, Alexander J, Christopher E, et al. Relationship of depression to increased risk of mortality and rehospitalization in patients with congestive heart failure. Arch Intern Med 2001;161:1849–56.

28. Gottlieb SS, Khatta M, Friedmann E, et al. The influence of age, gender, and race on the prevalence of depression in heart failure patients. J Am Coll Cardiol 2004;43:1542–9.

29. Morgan AL, Masoudi FA, Havranek EP, et al. Difficulty taking medications, depression, and health status in heart failure patients. J Card Fail 2006;12: 54–60.

30. Gehi A, Haas D, Pipkin S, et al. Depression and medication adherence in outpatients with coronary heart disease: findings from the Heart and Soul Study. Arch Intern Med 2005;165:2508–13.

31. Callahan CM, Hendrie HC, Tierney WM. Documentation and evaluation of cognitive impairment in elderly primary care patients. Ann Intern Med 1995;122: 422–9.

32. Pressler SJ. Cognitive functioning and chronic heart failure: a review of the literature (2002-July 2007). J Cardiovasc Nurs 2008;23:239–49.

33. Bennett SJ, Sauve MJ. Cognitive deficits in patients with heart failure: a review of the literature. J Cardiovasc Nurs 2003;18:219–42.

34. Dickson VV, Deatrick JA, Riegel B. A typology of heart failure self-care management in non-elders. Eur J Cardiovasc Nurs 2008;7:171–81.

35. Alves TC, Rays J, Fraguas R Jr, et al. Localized cerebral blood flow reductions in patients with heart failure: a study using 99mTc-HMPAO SPECT. J Neuroimaging 2005;15:150–6.

36. Woo MA, Kumar R, Macey PM, et al. Brain injury in autonomic, emotional, and cognitive regulatory areas in patients with heart failure. J Card Fail 2009;15:214–23.

37. Pullicino PM, Hart J. Cognitive impairment in congestive heart failure? Embolism vs hypoperfusion. Neurology 2001;57:1945–6.

38. Kalaria VG, Passannante MR, Shah T, et al. Effect of mitral regurgitation on left ventricular thrombus formation in dilated cardiomyopathy. Am Heart J 1998;135:215–20.

39. Loh E, Sutton MS, Wun CC, et al. Ventricular dysfunction and the risk of stroke after myocardial infarction. N Engl J Med 1997;336:251–7.

40. Georgiadis D, Sievert M, Cencetti S, et al. Cerebrovascular reactivity is impaired in patients with cardiac failure. Eur Heart J 2000;21:407–13.

41. Piette JD, Heisler M, Wagner TH. Cost-related medication underuse among chronically ill adults: the treatments people forgo, how often, and who is at risk. Am J Public Health 2004;94:1782–7.

42. Patterson ME, Blalock SJ, Smith AJ, et al. Associations between prescription copayment levels and beta-blocker medication adherence in commercially insured heart failure patients 50 years and older. Clin Ther 2011;33:608–16.

43. Dunlay SM, Eveleth JM, Shah ND, et al. Medication adherence among community-dwelling patients with heart failure. Mayo Clin Proc 2011;86:273–81.

44. Jaarsma T, Halfens R, Tan F, et al. Self-care and quality of life in patients with advanced heart failure: the effect of a supportive educational intervention. Heart Lung 2000;29:319–30.

45. Harrison MB, Browne GB, Roberts J, et al. Quality of life of individuals with heart failure: a randomized trial of the effectiveness of two models of hospital-to-home transition. Med Care 2002;40:271–82.

46. Wright SP, Walsh H, Ingley KM, et al. Uptake of self-management strategies in a heart failure management programme. Eur J Heart Fail 2003;5:371–80.

47. Prasun MA, Kocheril AG, Klass PH, et al. The effects of a sliding scale diuretic titration protocol in patients with heart failure. J Cardiovasc Nurs 2005;20:62–70.

48. Powell LH, Calvin JE Jr, Richardson D, et al. Self-management counseling in patients with heart failure: the heart failure adherence and retention randomized behavioral trial. JAMA 2010;304:1331–8.

49. Goldberg LR, Piette JD, Walsh MN, et al. Randomized trial of a daily electronic home monitoring system in patients with advanced heart failure: the Weight Monitoring in Heart Failure (WHARF) trial. Am Heart J 2003;146:705–12.

50. Hershberger RE, Ni H, Nauman DJ, et al. Prospective evaluation of an outpatient heart failure management program. J Card Fail 2001;7:64–74.

Effectiveness of Implantable Cardioverter Defibrillators and Cardiac Resynchronization Therapy in Heart Failure

James V. Freeman, MD, MPH, MS[a],*,
Frederick A. Masoudi, MD, MSPH[b]

KEYWORDS

- Sudden cardiac death • Implantable cardioverter-defibrillator • ICD
- Cardiac resynchronization therapy • CRT

KEY POINTS

- Implantable cardioverter defibrillators and cardiac resynchronization therapy with and without defibrillat or capability represent important and effective treatment modalities for select patients with HF.
- Additional investigation is required to better determine which patient populations most benefit from these cardiac devices and which device, implanting physician, and hospital characteristics optimize outcomes with these cardiac devices.

INTRODUCTION

The prevalence of heart failure (HF) has been steadily increasing. In 2006 there were approximately 5.8 million people with HF in the United States,[1] and an estimated 23 million people with HF worldwide.[2] Patients with HF carry a fivefold increased risk of sudden cardiac death (SCD)[3]; published series suggest that approximately 30% to 50% of all cardiac deaths in patients with HF are attributable to SCD.[3–8] Randomized trials over the past 15 years have shown mortality is reduced by implantable cardioverter defibrillator (ICD) implantation either for primary prevention of SCD in patients with HF and left ventricular systolic dysfunction (LVSD)[9–15] or secondary prevention in patients with a history of prior ventricular arrhythmias or aborted SCD (**Table 1**).[16–18] Other trials have demonstrated that cardiac resynchronization therapy improves quality of life and lowers rates of HF hospitalization in patients with symptomatic HF, LVSD, and a prolonged QRS complex already receiving optimal medical management; recent trial results have also suggested a mortality benefit with cardiac resynchronization therapy (CRT) in this population (**Table 2**).[15,19–33] Accordingly, US and international society clinical guidelines have supported the use of ICDs, CRT with pacemaker (CRT-P), and CRT with defibrillation function (CRT-D) for select patient populations

Funding Support: Dr Freeman is supported by an American Heart Association Pharmaceutical Round Table Outcomes Research Postdoctoral Fellowship (0875162N).
Disclosures: Dr Freeman has nothing to disclose; Dr Masoudi has grant funding from NHBLI and AHRQ; previous contract with Axio Research (blinded end point adjudication for a study sponsored by Affymax, Inc.); and contracts with the American College of Cardiology Foundation; the American Heart Association; and the Oklahoma Foundation for Medical Quality.
[a] Division of Cardiovascular Medicine, Stanford University School of Medicine, 300 Pasteur Drive, Falk Building, CVRC 5406, Stanford, CA 94305-5406, USA; [b] Division of Cardiology, University of Colorado Denver, Leprino Building, Room 522, Mail Stop B132, PO Box 6508, Aurora, CO 80045-0508, USA
* Corresponding author.
E-mail address: jfreeman@stanford.edu

Heart Failure Clin 9 (2013) 59–77
http://dx.doi.org/10.1016/j.hfc.2012.09.006
1551-7136/13/$ – see front matter © 2013 Elsevier Inc. All rights reserved.

heartfailure.theclinics.com

Table 1
Major randomized clinical trials of ICD therapy

Study	Year	Inclusion Criteria	Patients, n	ICD, n	Follow-up, mo	Main Result
Primary prevention in ischemic cardiomyopathy						
MADIT	1996	EF ≤35%, MI ≥3 weeks before entry, NSVT, inducible sustained VT on EPS, NYHA I–III	196	95	27	ICD therapy resulted in 54% RR reduction in mortality (95% CI 18%–74%), $P = .009$
CABG Patch	1997	EF ≤35%, abnormal SAECG, epicardial ICD during CABG	900	446	32	ICD therapy did not reduce mortality, $P = .64$
MUSTT	1999	EF ≤40%, MI ≥1 month before entry, asymptomatic NSVT	704	161	39 (median)	ICD therapy resulted in 55% RR reduction in mortality (95% CI 37%–68%), $P = .001$
MADIT II	2002	EF ≤30%, MI ≥1 month before entry, NYHA I–III	1232	742	20	ICD therapy resulted in 31% RR reduction in mortality (95% CI 7%–49%), $P = .016$
SCD-HeFT	2005	EF ≤35%, 3 months optimal medical therapy, NYHA II–III	2521 total, 1310 ischemic	829 total, 431 ischemic	45.5 (median)	Overall, ICD therapy resulted in 23% RR reduction in mortality (95% CI 4%–38%), $P = .007$; in ischemic patients ICD therapy resulted in nonsignificant 21% RR reduction in mortality (95% CI −4%–40%), $P = .05$. No evidence of effect modification by etiology.
Primary prevention in ischemic cardiomyopathy early after MI						
DINAMIT	2004	EF ≤35%, within 6–40 days of MI, depressed HRV or average Holter HR ≥80 bpm, NYHA I–III	674	332	33	ICD therapy did not reduce mortality, $P = .66$
IRIS	2009	EF ≤40%, within 5–31, HR ≥90 bpm or NSVT ≥150 bpm, NYHA I–III	898	445	37	ICD therapy did not reduce mortality, $P = .78$
Primary prevention in nonischemic cardiomyopathy						
CAT	2002	EF ≤30%, new onset DCM, NYHA II–III	104	50	66	ICD therapy did not reduce mortality, $P = .55$

AMIOVIRT	2003	EF ≤35%, DCM, asymptomatic NSVT, NYHA I–III	103	51	36	ICD therapy did not reduce mortality, $P = .80$
DEFINITE	2004	EF ≤35%, NSVT, NYHA I–III	458	229	29	ICD therapy resulted in nonsignificant 35% RR reduction in mortality (95% CI −6%–60%), $P = .08$
SCD-HeFT	2005	EF ≤35%, 3 months optimal medical therapy, NYHA II–III	2521 total, 1211 nonischemic	829 total, 398 nonischemic	45.5 (median)	Overall, ICD therapy resulted in 23% RR reduction in mortality (95% CI 4%–38%), $P = .007$; in nonischemic patients ICD therapy resulted in nonsignificant 27% RR reduction in mortality (95% CI −7%–50%), $P = .06$. No evidence of effect modification by etiology.
Secondary prevention						
AVID	1997	Any of: (1) VF, (2) VT with syncope, or (3) VT with severe symptoms and EF ≤40%	1016	507	18	ICD therapy resulted in 31% RR reduction in mortality (95% CI 10%–52%), $P = .02$
CASH	2000	Cardiac arrest secondary to ventricular arrhythmia	288	99	57	ICD therapy resulted in nonsignificant 23% RR reduction in mortality (97.5% CI lower bound −11%), 1-sided $P = .08$
CIDS	2000	Any of: (1) VF, (2) out-of-hospital cardiac arrest requiring defibrillation or cardioversion, (3) VT with syncope, (4) VT ≥150 bpm with symptoms and EF ≤35%, or (5) unmonitored syncope with subsequent VT	659	328	36	ICD therapy resulted in nonsignificant 20% RR reduction in mortality (95% CI −8%–40%), $P = .142$

Abbreviations: AMIOVIRT, Amiodarone versus Implantable Defibrillator Randomized Trial; AVID, Antiarrhythmic Drug versus Defibrillator; CABG, coronary artery bypass surgery; CABG Patch, Coronary Artery Bypass Graft Patch trial; CASH, Cardiac Arrest Survival in Hamburg; CAT, Cardiomyopathy Trial; CIDS, Canadian Implantable Defibrillator Study; DCM, dilated cardiomyopathy; DEFINITE, Defibrillators in Non-Ischemic Cardiomyopathy Treatment Evaluation; DINAMIT, Defibrillator in Acute Myocardial Infarction Trial; EF, ejection fraction; EPS, electrophysiology study; ICD, implantable cardioverter defibrillator; IRIS, Immediate Risk Stratification Improves Survival; MADIT, Multicenter Automatic Defibrillator Implantation Trial; MI, myocardial infarction; MUSTT, Multicenter Unsustained Tachycardia Trial Investigators; NSVT, nonsustained ventricular tachycardia; NYHA, New York Heart Association; RR, relative risk; SAECG, signal averaged ECG; SCD-HeFT, Sudden Cardiac Death in Heart Failure Trial; VF, ventricular fibrillation; VT, ventricular tachycardia.

Table 2
Major randomized clinical trials of CRT/CRT-D therapy

Study	Year	Inclusion Criteria	Patients, n	CRT/CRT-D, n	Follow-up, mo	Main Result
Primary prevention in moderate to severe heart failure comparing CRT with medical therapy						
MIRACLE	2002	EF ≤35%, NYHA III–IV, LVEDD ≥55 mm, QRS ≥130 ms, 6-minute walk ≤450 m	453	228 CRT	6	CRT therapy resulted in a 40% RR reduction in composite of death or HF hospitalization (95% CI 4%–63%), P = .03
COMPANION	2004	EF ≤35%, NYHA III–IV, on optimal medical therapy QRS ≥120 ms, PR > 150 ms, SR, hospitalization for HF in preceding 12 months	1520	617 CRT	16	CRT resulted in a 19% RR reduction in composite of death or hospitalization (95% CI 4%–31%), P = .014 and nonsignificant 24% RR reduction in death (95% CI −1%–42%), P = .06
CARE-HF	2005	EF ≤35%, NYHA III–IV despite optimal medical therapy, LVEDD ≥30 mm, QRS ≥150 ms or 120–149 ms with dyssynchrony	813	409 CRT	29	CRT therapy resulted in a 37% RR reduction in composite of death or unplanned hospitalization for cardiovascular event (95% CI 23%–49%), P<.001 and a 36% RR reduction in mortality (95% CI 15%–52%), P<.002
Primary prevention in moderate to severe heart failure comparing CRT-D to ICD or medical therapy						
MIRACLE ICD	2003	EF ≤35%, NYHA III–IV, stable medical therapy ≥1 month, LVEDD ≥55 mm, QRS ≥130 ms	369	187 CRT-D	6	CRT-D therapy did not reduce a composite of death or HF hospitalization, P = .69, or mortality alone, P = .96 (compared with ICD alone)
VENTAK CHF/ CONTAK CD	2003	EF ≤35%, NYHA II–IV, QRS ≥120 ms, stable medical therapy for 30 days	490	245 CRT-D	6	CRT-D therapy resulted in a nonsignificant 15% RR reduction in a composite of all-cause mortality, hospitalization for worsening HF, and ventricular tachyarrhythmias, P = .35 (compared with ICD alone)

COMPANION	2004	EF ≤35%, NYHA III–IV, on optimal medical therapy QRS ≥120 ms, PR > 150 ms, SR, hospitalization for HF in preceding 12 months	1520	595 CRT-D	16	CRT resulted in a 20% RR reduction in composite of death or hospitalization (95% CI 5%–32%), P = .011 and 36% RR reduction in death (95% CI 14%–52%), P = .003 (compared with medical therapy)
Primary prevention in mildly symptomatic heart failure comparing CRT to medical therapy or CRT-D to ICD						
REVERSE	2008	EF ≤40%, NYHA I–II, on optimal medical therapy for ≥3 mo, LVEDD ≥55 mm, QRS ≥120 ms, PR > 150 ms, SR	610	419 CRT and CRT-D	12	CRT resulted in nonsignificant 24% RR risk reduction in worsening on clinical composite response scale, P = .10, and a 53% RR reduction in time to first heart failure hospitalization, P = .03 (compared with CRT off)
MADIT-CRT	2009	EF ≤30%, NYHA I–II for ischemic and NYHA II for nonischemic, QRS ≥130 ms	1820	1089 CRT-D	29	CRT resulted in 34% RR reduction in death or nonfatal HF event (95% CI 16%–48%), P = .001, and no reduction in RR of death, P = .99 (compared with ICD only)
RAFT	2010	EF ≤30%, NYHA II–III, on optimal medical therapy QRS ≥120 ms or paced QRS ≥200 ms, SR or AF/AFL with good rate control or planned AVJ ablation	1798	894 CRT-D	40	CRT resulted in a 25% RR reduction in death or HF hospitalization (95% CI 13%–36%), P<.001, and 25% RR reduction in death (95% CI 9%–38%), P = .003 (compared with ICD only)

Abbreviations: AF, atrial fibrillation; AFL, atrial flutter; AVJ, atrioventricular junction; COMPANION, Comparison of Medical Therapy, Pacing, and Defibrillation in Heart Failure; CARE-HF, Cardiac Resynchronization- Heart Failure; CRT, cardiac resynchronization therapy; CRT-D, cardiac resynchronization therapy with defibrillator function; EF, ejection fraction; HF, heart failure; MADIT-CRT, Multicenter Automatic Defibrillator Implantation Trial- Cardiac Resynchronization Therapy; MIRACLE, Multicenter InSync Randomized Clinical Evaluation; MIRACLE ICD, Multicenter InSync ICD Randomized Clinical Evaluation; NYHA, New York Heart Association; RAFT, Resynchronization–Defibrillation for Ambulatory Heart Failure Trial; REVERSE, REsynchronization reVErses Remodeling in Systolic Left vEntricular Dysfunction; RR, relative risk; SR, sinus rhythm; VENTAK CHF/CONTAK CD, Cardiac Resynchronization Therapy for the Treatment of Heart Failure in Patients with Intraventricular Conduction Delay and Malignant Ventricular Tachyarrhythmias trial.

with HF.[34,35] Observational research has suggested that the effectiveness of ICD and CRT therapy may vary significantly depending on the characteristics of the patient, the characteristics of the device, the implanting physician, and the implanting hospital. These issues may increasingly influence device implantation practice.

CLINICAL TRIALS EVALUATING ICD THERAPY FOR PRIMARY PREVENTION OF SCD IN ISCHEMIC HF

HF can be attributable to a wide range of pathophysiological processes, including coronary artery disease (CAD). Indeed, patients with HF caused by CAD—ischemic cardiomyopathy—have a particularly high risk of SCD. Several clinical trials have demonstrated that prophylactic ICD implantation for the primary prevention of SCD reduces mortality in selected patients with ischemic cardiomyopathy. The indications for ICD implantation in current guidelines are largely derived from the inclusion criteria of the major clinical trials.

The first of these major trials was the MADIT trial (Multicenter Automatic Defibrillator Implantation Trial), which randomized 196 patients with a prior myocardial infarction (MI), nonsustained ventricular tachycardia (NSVT) on ambulatory monitoring, left ventricular ejection fraction (LVEF) less than 35%, and inducible sustained ventricular tachycardia (VT) during electrophysiology study (EPS) to prophylactic ICD or medical therapy alone.[9,13] After 27 months, those treated with an ICD had significantly lower total mortality (15 vs 39 deaths in the medical therapy group, hazard ratio [HR] 0.46, 95% confidence intervals [CI] 0.26–0.82, $P = .009$), as well as lower rates of cardiac death and SCD.

The MUSTT trial (Multicenter Unsustained Tachycardia Trial Investigators)[13] randomized 704 patients with a prior MI (≥ 1 month prior), asymptomatic NSVT, and LVEF of 40% or less to placebo or EPS-guided medical therapy with ICD after failure of at least one medical agent. There was a lower risk of cardiac arrest or death from arrhythmia among those receiving EPS-guided therapy (25% vs 32% without therapy, relative risk [RR] 0.73; 95% CI 0.53–0.99), which was largely attributed to ICD therapy in many of these patients (RR 0.24 for ICD vs without, 95% CI 0.13–0.45, $P<.001$). These findings therefore corroborated the findings of the MADIT study, but because MUSTT was not a trial of ICD therapy per se, further investigation with large trials that focused specifically on the efficacy of ICDs was warranted.

The MADIT II trial sought to confirm the findings of MADIT and MUSTT in a broader population.

This study randomized 1232 patients with an MI more than 30 days before enrollment and an LVEF of 30% or less to a prophylactic ICD or medical therapy.[11] Unlike MADIT-I, nonsustained VT was not a precondition of enrollment and routine EP testing for inducible VT was not performed. During a mean follow-up of 20 months, the mortality rates were significantly lower in the ICD group (14.2% vs 19.8% in the medical therapy group, HR 0.69, 95% CI 0.51–0.93, $P = .016$).

The largest of the primary prevention ICD trials published was the Sudden Cardiac Death in Heart Failure Trial (SCD-HeFT), which broadened inclusion to patients with nonischemic cardiomyopathy (discussed further later in this article).[14] SCD-HeFT included 2521 patients with an LVEF of 35% or less (48% ischemic) and New York Heart Association (NYHA) class II or III HF, and at a median follow-up of 45.5 months, there was significantly lower mortality in the ICD group (29% vs 22% in the placebo group, HR 0.77, 97.5% CI 0.62–0.96, $P = .007$). In a prespecified subgroup analysis of patients with ischemic cardiomyopathy for interaction, there was no evidence that the etiology of the cardiomyopathy modified the effect of ICDs on mortality. This study also identified no adverse consequences of ICD therapy on quality of life.[36]

Theuns and colleagues[37] performed a meta-analysis of ICD therapy for primary prevention of SCD in patients with ischemic cardiomyopathy. After considering trial heterogeneity and quality, their analysis focused on the MADIT, MADIT II, and SCD-HeFT trials. This pooled analysis showed significant reductions in all-cause mortality with RR reductions ranging from 22% to 59%. The pooled results using a random-effects model showed a 33% RR reduction in all-cause mortality with ICD therapy (95% CI 12%–49%, $P = .004$).

CLINICAL TRIALS EVALUATING ICD THERAPY FOR PRIMARY PREVENTION OF SCD IN HF EARLY AFTER MI OR CORONARY REVASCULARIZATION

All of the patients in the MADIT trials, and most of those in MUSTT and SCD-HeFT, were enrolled at least 3 weeks after an MI. Two subsequent trials evaluated the role of prophylactic ICD implantation in the first weeks following MI.

The DINAMIT trial (Defibrillator in Acute Myocardial Infarction Trial) randomized 674 patients with an MI within the preceding 6 to 40 days (mean 18 days), LVEF of 35% or less, and impaired cardiac autonomic function (manifested as depressed heart-rate variability or an average 24-hour heart rate on Holter monitoring ≥ 80 beats per minute) to ICD or medical therapy alone.[38]

During a mean follow-up period of 30 months, there was no difference in overall mortality between the 2 treatment groups (62 deaths vs 58 deaths in the control group, HR 1.08, 95% CI 0.76–1.55, P = .66). There were fewer deaths attributable to arrhythmia in the ICD group as compared with the control group (12 vs 29 in the control group, HR 0.42, 95% CI 0.22–0.83, P = .009), but more deaths from nonarrhythmic causes (50 vs 29 in the control group, HR 1.75; 95% CI 1.11–2.76, P = .02).

The more recent Immediate Risk Stratification Improves Survival (IRIS) trial randomized 898 patients with an MI within the preceding 5 to 31 days, and either LVEF of 40% or less and a resting heart rate of 90 or more beats per minute or NSVT of 150 or more beats per minute during Holter monitoring to ICD or medical therapy.[39] During a mean follow-up of 37 months, overall mortality was not reduced in the ICD group (116 vs 117 deaths in the control group, HR 1.04, 95% CI 0.81–1.35, P = .78). As with DINAMIT, there were fewer SCDs in the ICD group (27 vs 60 in the control group, HR 0.55, 95% CI 0.31–1.00, P = .049), but the number of non-SCDs was higher (68 vs 39 in the control group, HR 1.92, 95% CI 1.29–2.84, P = .001).

Despite the findings of DINAMIT and IRIS, a recent analysis of 111,707 ICD implants submitted to the National Cardiovascular Data Registry (NCDR) ICD Registry found that 9257 (8%) were implanted in patients within 40 days of an MI,[40] suggesting an ongoing gap between clinical practice and trial evidence.

There are number of possible reasons why DINAMIT and IRIS did not show the benefit from an ICD seen in the MADIT, MUSTT, and SCD-HeFT trials. A recent secondary analysis of DINAMIT showed that patients with ICDs who received appropriate defibrillator shock therapy had a relatively high burden of ischemic and heart failure events with a resulting high likelihood of nonarrhythmic death, which could negate the benefit of the ICD.[41,42] Patients who received appropriate shocks for ventricular arrhythmias had a fivefold increased risk of all-cause mortality.[41] Because of the relatively small size of the study, it is not clear whether this increased risk of nonarrhythmic death occurred as a result of risk inherent to the patients or as a result of ventricular arrhythmias or ICD shocks. It is also possible that ICD implantation might impose greater risk in patients immediately after acute MI than in those farther out from the event.[43] Finally, the enrollment requirements of reduced heart rate variability in DINAMIT and resting heart rate of 90 or more beats per minute in IRIS could

have selected a group of patients with a high risk of mortality from nonarrhythmic causes.[44]

The Coronary Artery Bypass Graft Patch trial sought to evaluate the efficacy of ICDs implanted at the time of revascularization. This trial randomized 900 patients with an LVEF of 35% or less and a positive signal-averaged electrocardiogram to medical therapy or epicardial ICD implantation at the time of coronary artery bypass surgery.[45] After a mean follow-up of 32 months, there was not a statistically significant difference in mortality (101 deaths vs 95 in the control group, HR 1.07, 95% CI 0.81–1.42; P = .64). This negative trial is the primary reason for the guideline recommendation against ICD implantation soon after coronary revascularization.[35]

CLINICAL TRIALS EVALUATING ICD THERAPY FOR PRIMARY PREVENTION OF SCD IN NONISCHEMIC HF

Although the risk of SCD in patients with nonischemic cardiomyopathies is not as high as that in those with an ischemic etiology, this risk remains substantially higher than the general population. Initial trials of ICD therapy for primary prevention in patients with nonischemic cardiomyopathy showed no survival benefit, but were limited by small sample size.[44,46] However, subsequent larger trials have demonstrated decreased mortality from prophylactic ICD implantation in this patient group.

The DEFINITE trial (Defibrillators in Non-Ischemic Cardiomyopathy Treatment Evaluation) randomized 458 patients with nonischemic dilated cardiomyopathy, LVEF 35% or less, and premature ventricular complexes or NSVT to treatment with medical therapy alone or medical therapy with a single-chamber ICD.[47] After a mean follow-up of 29 months, there was a trend toward lower mortality in the ICD group (28 vs 40 deaths in the medical therapy group, HR 0.65, 95% CI 0.40–1.06, P = .08) and a significantly lower risk of the secondary end point of SCD (3 vs 14 sudden deaths in the medical therapy group, HR 0.20, 95% CI 0.06–0.71, P = .006).

As described previously, the SCD-HeFT trial randomized 2521 (52% with nonischemic cardiomyopathy) to ICD therapy, amiodarone, or placebo.[14] In a prespecified subgroup analysis of patients with nonischemic cardiomyopathy for interaction, there was no evidence that the etiology of the cardiomyopathy modified the effect of ICDs on mortality. Thus, SCD-HeFT suggested that the relative benefits of ICDs are consistent in patients with both ischemic and nonischemic cardiomyopathy.

Desai and colleagues performed a meta-analysis of ICD implantation for primary prevention in patients with nonischemic cardiomyopathy that included 1854 patients from Cardiomyopathy Trial (CAT), Amiodarone versus Implantable Defibrillator Randomized Trial (AMIOVERT), DEFINITE, SCD-HeFT, and COMPANION (described later in this article).[48] This pooled analysis identified a significant reduction in all-cause mortality with an ICD compared with medical therapy (RR 0.69, 95% CI 0.55–0.87, P = .002). A more recent meta-analysis, including CAT, AMIOVERT, DEFINITE, and SCD-HeFT, showed a similar reduction in mortality risk (RR 0.74, 95% CI: 0.59–0.93; P = .009).[37]

CLINICAL TRIALS EVALUATING ICD THERAPY FOR SECONDARY PREVENTION OF SCD IN HF

A number of clinical trials have also evaluated the effectiveness of ICD therapy in patients after ventricular arrhythmia or aborted SCD (secondary prevention). Although not all of these trials exclusively enrolled patients with HF, most patients in the studies had symptomatic HF before their index cardiac arrest.

The largest study was the AVID trial (Antiarrhythmic Drug vs Defibrillator), which enrolled 1016 patients who were either (1) resuscitated from ventricular fibrillation arrest or (2) underwent cardioversion for sustained VT and had either syncope or other serious cardiac symptoms and an LVEF of 40% or less.[18] The trial was stopped when a significant survival benefit was identified in patients receiving the ICD compared with those treated with medical therapy (89% vs 82% at 1 year and 75% vs 65% at 3 years, P<.02). ICD-treated patients also had a lower risk of arrhythmic death (4.7% vs 10.8% with antiarrhythmic drugs).[49]

Two subsequent trials, the Cardiac Arrest Survival in Hamburg (CASH) and the Canadian Implantable Defibrillator Study (CIDS) were limited by small sample size but found nonsignificant trends toward lower mortality in patients who received ICDs for secondary prevention.[16,17] Fewer patients in these studies had symptomatic heart failure than in AVID. Thus, the populations of CASH and CIDS may have been at lower risk, further limiting their power to detect a difference between those treated with ICDs compared with those treated with medical therapy alone. Nonetheless, these studies did not contradict the finding in AVID that ICD therapy was effective for secondary prevention of ventricular arrhythmias and SCD.

Lee and colleagues[50] performed a meta-analysis of these 3 trials and a fourth smaller trial and found a significant 25% reduction in mortality with an ICD compared with medical therapy (HR 0.75, 95% CI 0.64–0.87, P = .0002). This effect was largely because of a 50% reduction in sudden death (hazard ratio 0.50, 95% CI 0.34–0.62).

SECONDARY ANALYSES OF RANDOMIZED CONTROLLED TRIALS AND OBSERVATIONAL STUDIES EVALUATING ICD THERAPY FOR PRIMARY PREVENTION IN HF SUBGROUPS

Secondary analyses of the randomized controlled trials (RCTs) described previously, as well as other observational studies, provide insights into the effectiveness of ICD therapy in patient subgroups, such as those with NYHA functional class IV HF, female sex, and older age. Most of these analyses have demonstrated a trend toward consistent effectiveness in these subgroups, although demonstration of statistical significance was often limited by sample size. Although these studies can be very informative, the small sample size of most of these studies and the nonrandomized nature of their design, with limited ability to control for unmeasured confounders, limits the strength of the evidence and the conclusiveness of the study results.

NYHA Functional Class IV

Patients with NYHA functional class IV HF that is refractory to medical therapy have a life expectancy that is generally less than 1 year, unless cardiac transplantation is performed or a ventricular assist device is placed. The role of ICD therapy for primary prevention of SCD in patients with NYHA class IV HF with a narrow QRS complex has not been studied in a randomized trial. However, a nonrandomized series of patients awaiting cardiac transplantation suggested a higher likelihood of survival to transplantation with ICD therapy, regardless of whether the ICD indication was well established.[51] The 2008 American College of Cardiology/American Heart Association/Heart Rhythm Society (ACC/AHA/HRS) guidelines recommend that ICD therapy is not indicated for NYHA class IV patients with drug-refractory congestive heart failure who are not candidates for cardiac transplantation or CRT-D (class III recommendation, see **Table 2; Table 3**). They further state that ICD therapy is not indicated for patients who do not have a reasonable expectation of survival with an acceptable functional status for at least 1 year, even if they meet ICD implantation criteria (class III recommendation). Given these considerations, for patients with NYHA class IV HF, an LVEF of 35% or less, and a narrow QRS complex who have a reasonable likelihood of survival for 1 year or longer or are awaiting cardiac transplantation, ICD therapy is often considered.

Women

Most patients included in the randomized trials that established the efficacy of ICDs were men. A meta-analysis was performed to study outcomes in women using pooled data from 5 RCTs of ICD implantation for the primary prevention of SCD in patients with HF and reduced LVEF (SCD-HeFT, MUSTT, MADIT II, DEFINITE, and DINAMIT).[52] The study found no significant difference in all-cause mortality between women receiving ICDs compared with those receiving medical therapy (HR 1.01; 95% CI 0.76–1.33). In addition, an analysis of 161,470 patients from the National Cardiovascular Data Registry (NCDR) ICD Registry showed that women were significantly more likely to experience an in-hospital adverse event associated with the procedure (4.4% vs 3.3%, OR 1.32, 95% CI 1.24–1.39).[53] Nonetheless, none of the 5 randomized trials used in the previously mentioned meta-analysis reported a significant interaction between sex and ICD therapy on overall mortality, and the current 2008 ACC/AHA/HRS guidelines and 2010 Heart Failure Society of America guidelines do not tailor recommendations by patient sex.

Older Persons and Patients with Multiple Coexisting Illnesses

Older adults and patients with major comorbidities have been underrepresented in major ICD trials. Because of the risks of noncardiac death, some older adults and those with multiple or severe comorbidities may be less likely to derive benefit from an ICD. A recent meta-analysis that included patients from MADIT II, DEFINITE, and SCD-HeFT, found that ICD implantation for primary prevention in patients with LVSD significantly lowered mortality in patients younger than 65 years (HR 0.65; 95% CI 0.50–0.83, P<.001); there was a nonsignificant trend toward lower mortality in patients 65 years or older (HR 0.81; 95% CI 0.62–1.05, P = .11).[54] Several observational studies have shown a significantly lower mortality with primary prevention ICDs in the elderly, however. A retrospective cohort study of the clinical effectiveness of ICDs was conducted in a cohort of 4685 Medicare beneficiaries (mean age 75.2 years) with HF and LVEF of 35% or less who received ICDs between 2003 and 2006.[55] Mortality was significantly lower among patients who received an ICD compared with those who did not (19.8% vs 27.6% at 1 year and 38.1% vs 52.3% at 3 years, HR 0.71, 95% CI 0.56–0.91, P<.001). Format testing for an

interaction between age and ICD therapy on mortality was not significant (P for interaction = .31). Chan and colleagues[56] performed a prospective cohort study of 965 patients with ischemic and nonischemic cardiomyopathies (LVEF ≤ 35%) and no prior ventricular arrhythmia. After a mean follow-up of 34 months, ICD therapy was associated with a 31% lower all-cause mortality (HR 0.69; 95% CI 0.50–0.96; P = .03); this relationship was consistent after stratification by age (<65, 65–74, and ≥75), ischemic etiology, ejection fraction (>25% vs ≤25%), and the presence of major comorbid conditions (probability values for all interactions >0.05). A recent analysis of 4566 patients from the Advancements in ICD Therapy (ACT) Registry showed that more than 40% of new ICDs and CRT-D devices were implanted in patients older than 70 and more than 10% in patients 80 years or older, suggesting that the elderly have not been excluded from receiving these cardiac devices in community practice.[57]

In contrast, patients with very severe comorbidities, such as severe chronic kidney disease, may not benefit from ICD implantation. A post hoc analysis from the MADIT II trial found no mortality benefit in patients with an estimated glomerular filtration rate less than 35 mL/min (mean 29 mL/min, no patient was on dialysis), whereas a benefit was noted in patients with better renal function.[58] This differential in ICD benefit may be at least partially explained by significantly higher rates of postprocedure complications. An analysis of 164,069 patients from the NCDR ICD Registry demonstrated that patients with end-stage renal disease (ESRD) (n = 6851, 4.4%) had higher rates of comorbid medical conditions, major complications, and total complications. Unadjusted in-hospital mortality was almost fivefold higher among patients with ESRD (1.9% vs 0.4%, P<.0001) and multivariable analysis confirmed that ESRD was independently associated with total in-hospital complications (odds ratio [OR] 1.38, 95% CI 1.23–1.54, P<.0001).[59]

SINGLE-LEAD VERSUS DUAL-LEAD ICDS

Many of the major clinical trials evaluating ICD efficacy, such as SCD-HeFT, included only single-chamber devices or relatively few dual-chamber devices, with the main exception being MADIT II, which implanted dual-chamber devices in approximately half the study participants.[11,14] However, currently in the United States approximately twice as many dual-chamber ICDs are placed as single-chamber devices,[60] despite limited evidence to suggest clinical benefit with the more complex and expensive devices. MADIT II found

Table 3
Guideline recommendations for ICD, CRT, and CRT-D therapy in patients with HF

Guideline	Recommendations
ICD therapy for primary prevention in patients with LVSD	
2008 ACC/AHA/HRS Guidelines for Device-Based Therapy of Cardiac Rhythm Abnormalities[35]	Ischemic cardiomyopathy: 1. LVEF ≤35%, MI ≥40 days prior, NYHA functional Class II or III. (Level of Evidence: A, Class I recommendation) 2. LVEF ≤30%, MI ≥40 days prior, NYHA functional Class I. (Level of Evidence: A, Class I recommendation) 3. LVEF ≤40%, NSVT due to prior MI, inducible VF or sustained VT at electrophysiology study. (Level of Evidence: B, Class I recommendation) 4. LVEF ≤35% and NYHA functional Class I can also be considered. (Level of Evidence: C, Class IIb recommendation) Nonischemic dilated cardiomyopathy: 1. LVEF ≤35% and NYHA functional class II or III. (Level of Evidence: B, Class I recommendation).
2009 Focused Update: ACCF/AHA Guidelines for the Diagnosis and Management of Heart Failure in Adults	1. Nonischemic dilated cardiomyopathy or ischemic heart disease ≥40 days post-MI, an LVEF ≤35%, and NYHA functional class II or III symptoms while receiving chronic optimal medical therapy with reasonable expectation of survival with a good functional status for >1 year. (Level of Evidence: A, Class I recommendation)
ICD therapy for secondary prevention[a]	
2008 ACC/AHA/HRS Guidelines for Device-Based Therapy of Cardiac Rhythm Abnormalities	1. Cardiac arrest attributable to VF or hemodynamically unstable sustained VT after evaluation to define the cause of the event and to exclude any completely reversible causes. (Level of Evidence: A, Class I recommendation) 2. Syncope of undetermined origin with clinically relevant, hemodynamically significant sustained VT or VF induced at electrophysiological study. (Level of Evidence: B, Class I recommendation)
2009 Focused Update: ACCF/AHA Guidelines for the Diagnosis and Management of Heart Failure in Adults	1. Current or prior symptoms of HF and reduced LVEF who have a history of cardiac arrest, VF, or hemodynamically destabilizing VT. (Level of Evidence: A, Class I recommendation)

CRT or CRT-D therapy

2008 ACC/AHA/HRS Guidelines for Device-Based Therapy of Cardiac Rhythm Abnormalities	1. LVEF ≤35%, QRS duration ≥0.12 seconds, sinus rhythm, NYHA functional Class III or ambulatory Class IV heart failure symptoms with optimal recommended medical therapy. (Level of Evidence: A, Class I recommendation)
	2. LVEF ≤35%, QRS duration ≥0.12 seconds, atrial fibrillation, NYHA functional Class III or ambulatory Class IV heart failure symptoms on optimal recommended medical therapy. (Level of Evidence: B, Class IIa recommendation)
	3. LVEF ≤35% with NYHA functional Class III or ambulatory Class IV symptoms who are receiving optimal recommended medical therapy and who have frequent dependence on ventricular pacing, CRT is reasonable. (Level of Evidence: C, Class IIa recommendation)
	4. LVEF ≤35% with NYHA functional Class I or II symptoms who are receiving optimal recommended medical therapy and who are undergoing implantation of a permanent pacemaker and/or ICD with anticipated frequent ventricular pacing, CRT may be considered. (Level of Evidence: C, Class IIb recommendation)
2009 Focused Update: ACCF/AHA Guidelines for the Diagnosis and Management of Heart Failure in Adults	1. LVEF ≤35%, sinus rhythm, NYHA functional class III or ambulatory class IV symptoms despite recommended, optimal medical therapy and who have cardiac dyssynchrony, which is currently defined as a QRS duration ≥0.12 seconds, unless contraindicated. (Level of Evidence: A, Class I recommendation)
	2. LVEF ≤35%, a QRS duration ≥0.12 seconds, atrial fibrillation, NYHA functional class III or ambulatory class IV heart failure symptoms on optimal recommended medical therapy. (Level of Evidence: B, Class IIa recommendation)
	3. LVEF ≤35% with NYHA functional class III or ambulatory class IV symptoms who are receiving optimal recommended medical therapy and who have frequent dependence on ventricular pacing, CRT is reasonable. (Level of Evidence: C, Class IIa recommendation)

Abbreviations: ACC, American College of Cardiology; ACCF, American College of Cardiology Foundation; CRT, cardiac resynchronization therapy; AHA, American Heart Association; HF, heart failure; HRS, Heart Rhythm Society; ICD, implantable cardioverter defibrillator; LVEF, left ventricular ejection fraction; LVSD, left ventricular systolic dysfunction; MI, myocardial infarction; NYHA, New York Heart Association; VF, ventricular fibrillation; VT, ventricular tachycardia.

[a] Currently the guidelines do not distinguish between patients with and without clinical HF with regard to indications for ICD implantation for secondary prevention of SCD.

Data from Epstein AE, DiMarco JP, Ellenbogen KA, et al. ACC/AHA/HRS 2008 guidelines for device-based therapy of cardiac rhythm abnormalities: a report of the American College of Cardiology/American Heart Association Task Force on Practice Guidelines (Writing Committee to revise the ACC/AHA/NASPE 2002 guideline update for implantation of cardiac pacemakers and antiarrhythmia devices): developed in collaboration with the American Association for Thoracic Surgery and Society of Thoracic Surgeons. Circulation 2008;117(21):e350–408; and Jessup M, Abraham WT, Casey DE, et al. 2009 focused update: ACCF/AHA guidelines for the diagnosis and management of heart failure in adults: a report of the American College of Cardiology Foundation/American Heart Association Task Force on Practice Guidelines: developed in collaboration with the International Society for Heart and Lung Transplantation. Circulation 2009;119(14):1977–2016.

no differences in survival between single-lead and dual-lead devices; a post hoc analysis found no survival advantage of a dual-chamber device following heart failure hospitalization.[12] Several other early studies reported small or even nonexistent advantages of dual-chamber arrhythmia discrimination[61–63]; however, more recent studies have suggested a benefit of dual-chamber devices over single-chamber devices.[64–66] To resolve this issue, Theuns and colleagues[67] performed a meta-analysis of 5 randomized controlled studies: the 1 + 1 Trial,[65] the Prevention of INAPPropriate Therapy study,[63] (PINAPPs), the Detect Supra-Ventricular Tachycardia (Detect SVT) study,[66] a study by Deisenhofer and colleagues,[62] and a study by Kuhlkamp and colleagues.[61] The meta-analysis included 748 patients (380 with single-chamber and 368 patients with dual-chamber). Dual-chamber arrhythmia discrimination was not associated with a significant reduction in the number of patients who received inappropriate therapy relative to single-chamber discrimination (OR 0.97, 95% CI 0.68–1.38, $P = .85$). A second analysis that excluded the 1 + 1 Trial owing to evidence of statistical heterogeneity confirmed this finding (OR 1.18, 95% CI 0.83–1.81, $P = .31$). Thus, current evidence suggests little incremental benefit to the use of dual-chamber over single-chamber ICDs, but clinical practice still favors the more complicated and expensive devices.

OBSERVATIONAL STUDIES EVALUATING ICD-RELATED COMPLICATIONS

Complications attributable to ICD implantation in clinical trials generally decreased with successive trials and varied because of disparate definitions of complications between trials. The NCDR ICD Registry was initiated in 2006 and requires hospitals to submit in-hospital data for ICD implantations for primary prevention among Medicare patients, although 80% of hospitals submit data on all ICD implantations performed, irrespective of the payer or clinical indication. A number of observational studies performed using the registry data have greatly improved our understanding of ICD procedure complications in recent community practice, including the studies demonstrating higher complication rates among women and patients with ESRD described previously.[53,59] In addition, Curtis and colleagues[68] studied 111,293 ICD implantations and demonstrated that complication rates were increased when the device was implanted by nonelectrophysiologist cardiologists (RR 1.11 compared with electrophysiologists, 95% CI, 1.01–1.21) or thoracic surgeons (RR 1.44 compared with electrophysiologists, 95% CI 1.15–1.79). A subsequent NCDR study then demonstrated that patients who have an ICD implanted at a high-volume hospital are less likely to have an adverse event associated with the procedure than patients who have an ICD implanted at a low-volume hospital.[60] These studies therefore suggest that implanting physician and hospital characteristics may significantly affect patient outcomes after ICD placement.

CLINICAL TRIAL EVALUATING CARDIAC RESYNCHRONIZATION THERAPY IN MODERATE TO SEVERE HF

CRT is the pacing of both cardiac ventricles to synchronize ventricular contraction and optimize cardiac output. CRT can be achieved with a device designed only for pacing (CRT-P) or can be incorporated into a combination device with an ICD (CRT-D). CRT has been evaluated in patients with moderate to severe HF in a number of randomized trials over the past 15 years. Early studies showed a clinical benefit with CRT, largely owing to symptom reduction, but these studies were limited by small sample size and modest follow-up duration. Since 2002, a number of large, longer-term clinical trials have been published that evaluated the clinical benefit of CRT with and without defibrillator capability for the reduction of symptoms, hospitalizations, and mortality.

The earliest of these studies was the MIRACLE trial (Multicenter InSync Randomized Clinical Evaluation),[24] which randomized 453 patients with moderate to severe heart failure, decreased LVEF, and prolonged QRS to medical therapy or CRT; after 6 months of follow-up, patients with a CRT had significantly greater improvements in 6-minute walk distance, NYHA functional class, quality of life, exercise treadmill testing time, and LVEF. Perhaps more importantly, patients treated with CRT had a significantly lower rate of HF hospitalization (34 vs 18 in the CRT group, HR 0.5; 95% CI 0.28–0.88, $P = .02$), and also a trend toward lower mortality (16 vs 12 in the CRT group, HR 0.73; 95% CI 0.34–1.54, $P = .40$).

Two large trials were therefore performed to corroborate the findings in MIRACLE. The COMPANION trial (Comparison of Medical Therapy, Pacing, and Defibrillation in Heart Failure) randomly assigned 1520 patients with NYHA class III–IV heart failure, a QRS interval of 120 ms or longer, and LVEF of 35% or less to receive optimal pharmacologic therapy alone (diuretics, angiotensin-converting enzyme inhibitors, beta-blockers, and spironolactone) or in combination with CRT-P or CRT-D.[15,22] There was a nearly significant improvement in all-cause mortality in the CRT-D group (12% vs 19% in the medical therapy group, HR 0.64, 95% CI 0.48–0.86) and the CRT-P group (15% vs 19%, HR 0.76, 95% CI 0.58–1.01). In addition, there was a nonsignificant trend toward decreased all-cause mortality for CRT-D compared with CRT-P (OR 0.79, 95% CI 0.60–1.06).[69] At 3 and 6 months, both CRT arms showed significant improvements in NYHA class, 6-minute walk distance, and systolic blood pressure compared with medical therapy alone. All-cause, cardiac, and HF hospitalization rates were significantly reduced in both CRT arms compared with medical therapy alone.[70] These results were particularly impressive given that during the course of the study, a large proportion of patients in the medical therapy arm of the trial withdrew to receive a device because of arrhythmia or HF (26%).

The CARE-HF trial (Cardiac Resynchronization–Heart Failure) randomized 813 patients with NYHA class III or IV HF (62% nonischemic), an LVEF of 35% or less (median 25%), and QRS prolongation (≥120 ms) to CRT-P and medical therapy or medical therapy alone.[21,23] At a mean follow-up of 29 months, the investigators found a significant reduction in the primary end point of time to death from any cause or unplanned hospitalization for a major cardiovascular event (39% vs 55% with medical therapy, HR 0.63, 95% CI 0.51–0.77, P<.001) and a significant reduction in the secondary end point of total mortality (20% vs 30%, HR 0.64, 95% CI 0.48–0.85, P<.002). At 90 days, there were significant improvements in quality of life and NYHA class. Thus, the CARE-HF study confirmed many of the findings of COMPANION and demonstrated more definitively the mortality benefit of CRT therapy in patients with moderate to severe HF.

McAlister and colleagues[71] published a meta-analysis of CRT efficacy that included a total of 14 randomized trials (4420 patients), including CARE-HF,[21,23] COMPANION,[15,22] MIRACLE and MIRACLE ICD (Multicenter InSync ICD Randomized Clinical Evaluation),[24–26] MUSTIC-SR and MUSTIC-AF (Multisite Stimulation in Cardiomyopathies),[27–29] PATH-CHF (Pacing Therapies in Congestive Heart Failure),[30] VENTAK CHF/CONTAK CD (Cardiac resynchronization therapy for the treatment of heart failure in patients with intraventricular conduction delay and malignant ventricular tachyarrhythmias trial),[31] and HOBI-PACE (Homburg Biventricular Pacing Evaluation).[32] All patients in the CRT studies had LV systolic dysfunction (mean LVEF range 21%–30%) and prolonged QRS duration (mean range, 155–209 ms), and 91% had NYHA class III or IV

HF symptoms despite optimal pharmacotherapy. The meta-analysis demonstrated a greater likelihood of improvement by at least 1 NYHA class between baseline and 6 months with CRT (59% vs 37%, RR 1.55, 95% CI 1.25–1.92) as well as improvements in LVEF (weighted mean difference, 3.0%, 95% CI 0.9%–5.1%), 6-minute walk test distance (weighted mean difference 24 m, 95% CI 13–35 m), and quality of life (weighted mean difference in Minnesota Living With Heart Failure Questionnaire, 8.0 points, 95% CI 5.6–10.4 points). The patients with CRT had lower rates of HF hospitalization (19% vs 27% in controls, RR 0.63, 95% CI 0.43–0.93), and all-cause mortality (13.2% vs 15.5% in controls, RR 0.78; 95% CI, 0.67–0.91). Using just trials that compared CRT-D with ICD therapy, CRT was associated with a trend toward lower mortality (RR 0.86; 95% CI 0.54–1.39).

CLINICAL TRIALS EVALUATING CRT IN PATIENTS WITH MILDLY SYMPTOMATIC HF

Other trials have evaluated the clinical benefit of CRT in patients with mild HF symptoms. The first of these studies was the REVERSE trial (REsynchronization reVErses Remodeling in Systolic left vEntricular dysfunction), which randomized 610 patients with NYHA functional class I or II HF, a QRS of 120 ms or longer, and an LVEF of 40% or less who received a CRT device (±defibrillator) to active CRT or control (CRT off).[33] After a 12-month follow-up, patients with CRT experienced less clinical heart failure deterioration on a composite index (P = .10), greater improvement in LV end-systolic volume index (–18.4 mL/m2 vs –1.3 mL/m2, P<.0001), and delayed time-to-first HF hospitalization (HR 0.47, P = .03). Thus, this study showed that CRT may improve patient clinical status even in those with mildly symptomatic heart failure, resulting in decreased hospitalization rates.

The REVERSE study was followed by 2 larger confirmatory trials. The MADIT-CRT trial (Multicenter Automatic Defibrillator Implantation Trial–Cardiac Resynchronization Therapy) randomly assigned 1820 patients with ischemic or nonischemic cardiomyopathy, an LVEF of 30% or less, a QRS duration of 130 ms or longer, and NYHA class I or II symptoms to receive CRT-D or ICD alone.[19] During an average follow-up of 2.4 years, CRT-D resulted in a significant decrease in the primary end point of death from any cause or a nonfatal HF event (17.2% vs 25.3% in the ICD group, HR 0.66; 95% CI 0.52–0.84, P = .001). There was no significant difference between the 2 groups in the overall risk of death (HR 1.0, 95% CI 0.69–1.44, P = .99) with a 3% annual mortality rate in each treatment group; thus, the differences in the primary end point were entirely accounted for by differences in HF events. The benefit did not differ significantly between patients with ischemic cardiomyopathy and those with nonischemic cardiomyopathy.

Most recently, the RAFT trial (Resynchronization–Defibrillation for Ambulatory Heart Failure Trial)[20] randomized 1798 patients with NYHA class II or III HF, LVEF of 30% or less, and an intrinsic QRS duration of 120 ms or longer or a paced QRS duration of 200 ms or longer to receive either an ICD alone or an ICD plus CRT (CRT-D). The study unexpectedly showed a lower mortality in the CRT-D group (186 deaths vs 236 deaths in the ICD group, HR 0.75, 95% CI 0.62–0.91, P = .003) in addition to fewer HF hospitalizations (174 vs 236 in the ICD group, HR 0.68, 95% CI 0.56–0.83, P<.001). Thus, the RAFT trial demonstrated both clinical improvement and mortality benefits from CRT-D compared with ICD alone in patients with mildly symptomatic HF.

A recent analysis from the NCDR ICD Registry demonstrated that 23.7% of CRT devices placed between January 2006 and June 2008 were placed without meeting all 3 implant criteria, most often owing to NYHA functional class below III (13.1% of implants) as well as QRS interval duration less than 120 ms (12.0%).[72] This suggests that community practice was proceeding with CRT implantation in less symptomatic patients before definitive trial evidence. Presumably, device use in this patient population is likely to increase in the future; however, given the limited available evidence, the use of this relatively expensive therapy should be evaluated carefully before it is adopted widely in patients with modest symptoms.

SECONDARY ANALYSES OF RCTS AND OBSERVATIONAL STUDIES EVALUATING CRT IN SUBGROUPS

Secondary analyses of the clinical trials and other observational studies have evaluated the effectiveness of CRT therapy in patient subgroups according to NYHA functional class, sex, and age. Most of these analyses have demonstrated a trend toward consistent effectiveness in these subgroups, although demonstration of statistical significance was generally limited by sample size.

NYHA Functional Class IV HF

Although patients with NYHA class IV HF were included in the previously mentioned clinical trials, most enrolled patients were NYHA class III, and, as with ICDs, it has been suggested that NYHA class IV patients may benefit less from CRT or CRT-D given the limited life expectancy of these patients. A retrospective analysis of the COMPANION trial addressed this issue.[73] Among the 1520 patients enrolled in COMPANION, 217 patients were classified as NYHA class IV. However, patients were excluded from the trial if they were expected to undergo cardiac transplantation within 6 months or had been hospitalized for HF within 30 days of entry. Thus, the 217 included patients represented a relatively stable, ambulatory class IV cohort. The investigators demonstrated that in the class IV patients, the primary end point of time to death or hospitalization for any cause was significantly improved by both CRT-P (HR 0.64, 95% CI 0.43–0.94, P = .02) and CRT-D (HR 0.62, 95% CI 0.42–0.90, P = .01). Time to all-cause death trended to an improvement in both CRT (HR 0.67, 95% CI 0.41–1.10, P = .11) and CRT-D (HR 0.63, 95% CI 0.39–1.03, P = .06). Time to SCD was also significantly reduced in the CRT-D group (HR 0.27, 95% CI 0.08–0.90, P = .03). Thus, at least in relatively stable patients with NYHA class IV, CRT-P and CRT-D do appear to offer significant clinical benefits.

Elderly and More Comorbid Patients

Randomized trials have not specifically addressed the benefit of CRT in elderly patients. However, in both CARE-HF and COMPANION, the mean age was approximately 65 years and the benefit from CRT was similar in patients older than and younger than the mean age.[15,21]

Women

The large CRT trials to date have included a relatively modest (15%–30%) percentage of women, and no studies have specifically evaluated the efficacy of CRT in women. Germany and Ripley,[74] however, conducted a review of the results of randomized CRT trials to evaluate if there was a differential effect in women and men. They found that none of these studies showed a significant difference in CRT effectiveness by sex, and a few small studies suggested a more positive effect in women. Thus, the available evidence suggests that CRT is at least if not more effective in women as it is in men.

Right Bundle Branch Block

The efficacy of CRT in patients with right bundle branch block (RBBB) is not established. Most patients in the controlled CRT trials had left bundle branch block (LBBB); RBBB was present in 15% or fewer of patients in most trials. A recent retrospective cohort study using the Medicare Implantable Cardioverter-Defibrillator Registry (2005–2006) merged with Medicare data on post-implantation survival and HF hospitalizations (n = 44,878) evaluated whether outcomes differed by QRS morphology.[75] Death (46% vs 35% with LBBB) and a combined end point of death or HF hospitalization (60% vs 50% with LBBB) were significantly more common in patients with RBBB in unadjusted survival analysis. In a proportional hazards regression analysis adjusted for other risk factors, the survival curves continued to separate during 4 years of follow-up between patients with RBBB compared with those with LBBB (1-year HR 1.44, 95% CI 1.26–1.65, $P<.0001$; 3-year HR 1.37, 95% CI 1.26–1.49, $P<.0001$). Similar Cox proportional-hazards models for the outcomes of mortality and a composite of death and HF hospitalization with the addition of interaction terms for BBB morphology and CRT implantation showed significant interaction ($P<.05$). This suggests that patients with RBBB may fair worse with CRT than patients with LBBB; however, the absolute survival benefit for this population remains unclear at this time. Thus, recommendations for CRT in the 2008 ACC/AHA/HRS guidelines do not specify QRS morphology criteria and state that there is not yet sufficient evidence to provide specific recommendations for patients with RBBB.

GUIDELINE RECOMMENDATIONS

Based on clinical trials and meta-analytic and observational studies, definitive recommendations regarding the use of ICD, CRT, and CRT-D therapy have been delineated in the 2008 ACC/AHA/HRS Guidelines for Device-Based Therapy of Cardiac Rhythm Abnormalities and the 2009 Focused Update: ACCF/AHA Guidelines for the Diagnosis and Management of Heart Failure in Adults (see **Table 3**).[35,76]

SUMMARY

Randomized trials and observational data have consistently demonstrated the benefit of ICDs for primary prevention of SCD in patients with HF and LVSD[9–15] or secondary prevention in patients with a history of prior ventricular arrhythmias or aborted SCD, most of whom have HF.[16–18] Secondary and post hoc analyses of trial data, as well as observational data, generally suggest that ICD therapy is effective in most selected subpopulations, such as the elderly and patients with NYHA class IV HF symptoms, but some studies suggest that ICDs may not be as effective

in women and those with severe comorbidities, such as ESRD. Although there is limited evidence for an incremental benefit achieved with dual-chamber compared with single-chamber ICDs, the former devices are placed almost twice as frequently in the United States. Finally, observational data have recently shown that ICD procedural outcomes are improved when the device is placed by an electrophysiologist and at a high-volume hospital.

More recently, clinical trials have demonstrated that cardiac resynchronization therapy improves quality of life and lowers rates of HF hospitalization in patients with symptomatic HF, LVSD, and a prolonged QRS complex already receiving optimal medical management; recent trial results have also suggested a mortality benefit with CRT in this population.[15,19–22] In addition, recent trial data suggest that CRT reduces nonfatal events among mildly symptomatic patients (NYHA class I–II); however, the cost-effectiveness of CRT in this population remains unclear. As with ICDs, secondary and post hoc analyses of trial data as well as observational data suggest that CRT remains effective in most selected subpopulations, including stable NYHA class IV patients, the very elderly, and women. Recent observational work has suggested that CRT may not benefit patients with an RBBB QRS morphology to the same extent as those with an LBBB pattern, although because more conclusive studies are currently lacking, the guidelines do not tailor the recommendations based on QRS morphology.

In summary, ICDs, CRT-P, and CRT-D represent important and effective treatment modalities for select patients with HF. Additional investigation is required to better determine which patient populations most benefit from these cardiac devices and which device, implanting physician, and hospital characteristics optimize outcomes with these cardiac devices.

REFERENCES

1. Lloyd-Jones D, Adams RJ, Brown TM, et al. Heart disease and stroke statistics—2010 update: a report from the American Heart Association. Circulation 2010;121(7):e46–215.
2. McMurray JJ, Petrie MC, Murdoch DR, et al. Clinical epidemiology of heart failure: public and private health burden. Eur Heart J 1998;19(Suppl P):P9–16.
3. Kannel WB, Wilson PW, D'Agostino RB, et al. Sudden coronary death in women. Am Heart J 1998;136(2):205–12.
4. Mosterd A, Cost B, Hoes AW, et al. The prognosis of heart failure in the general population: The Rotterdam Study. Eur Heart J 2001;22(15):1318–27.

5. Effect of enalapril on survival in patients with reduced left ventricular ejection fractions and congestive heart failure. The SOLVD Investigators. N Engl J Med 1991;325(5):293–302.

6. Effect of enalapril on mortality and the development of heart failure in asymptomatic patients with reduced left ventricular ejection fractions. The SOLVD Investigators. N Engl J Med 1992;327(10):685–91.

7. Effect of metoprolol CR/XL in chronic heart failure: Metoprolol CR/XL Randomised Intervention Trial in Congestive Heart Failure (MERIT-HF). Lancet 1999;353(9169):2001–7.

8. Pfeffer MA, Braunwald E, Moye LA, et al. Effect of captopril on mortality and morbidity in patients with left ventricular dysfunction after myocardial infarction. Results of the survival and ventricular enlargement trial. The SAVE Investigators. N Engl J Med 1992;327(10):669–77.

9. Moss AJ, Hall WJ, Cannom DS, et al. Improved survival with an implanted defibrillator in patients with coronary disease at high risk for ventricular arrhythmia. Multicenter Automatic Defibrillator Implantation Trial Investigators. N Engl J Med 1996;335(26):1933–40.

10. Moss AJ, Fadl Y, Zareba W, et al. Survival benefit with an implanted defibrillator in relation to mortality risk in chronic coronary heart disease. Am J Cardiol 2001;88(5):516–20.

11. Moss AJ, Zareba W, Hall WJ, et al. Prophylactic implantation of a defibrillator in patients with myocardial infarction and reduced ejection fraction. N Engl J Med 2002;346(12):877–83.

12. Greenberg H, Case RB, Moss AJ, et al. Analysis of mortality events in the Multicenter Automatic Defibrillator Implantation Trial (MADIT-II). J Am Coll Cardiol 2004;43(8):1459–65.

13. Buxton AE, Lee KL, Fisher JD, et al. A randomized study of the prevention of sudden death in patients with coronary artery disease. Multicenter Unsustained Tachycardia Trial Investigators. N Engl J Med 1999;341(25):1882–90.

14. Bardy GH, Lee KL, Mark DB, et al. Amiodarone or an implantable cardioverter-defibrillator for congestive heart failure. N Engl J Med 2005;352(3):225–37.

15. Bristow MR, Saxon LA, Boehmer J, et al. Cardiac-resynchronization therapy with or without an implantable defibrillator in advanced chronic heart failure. N Engl J Med 2004;350(21):2140–50.

16. Kuck KH, Cappato R, Siebels J, et al. Randomized comparison of antiarrhythmic drug therapy with implantable defibrillators in patients resuscitated from cardiac arrest: the Cardiac Arrest Study Hamburg (CASH). Circulation 2000;102(7):748–54.

17. Connolly SJ, Gent M, Roberts RS, et al. Canadian implantable defibrillator study (CIDS): a randomized trial of the implantable cardioverter defibrillator against amiodarone. Circulation 2000;101(11):1297–302.

18. A comparison of antiarrhythmic-drug therapy with implantable defibrillators in patients resuscitated from near-fatal ventricular arrhythmias. The Antiarrhythmics versus Implantable Defibrillators (AVID) Investigators. N Engl J Med 1997;337(22):1576–83.

19. Moss AJ, Hall WJ, Cannom DS, et al. Cardiac-resynchronization therapy for the prevention of heart-failure events. N Engl J Med 2009;361(14):1329–38.

20. Tang AS, Wells GA, Talajic M, et al. Cardiac-resynchronization therapy for mild-to-moderate heart failure. N Engl J Med 2010;363(25):2385–95.

21. Cleland JG, Daubert JC, Erdmann E, et al. The effect of cardiac resynchronization on morbidity and mortality in heart failure. N Engl J Med 2005;352(15):1539–49.

22. Saxon LA, Bristow MR, Boehmer J, et al. Predictors of sudden cardiac death and appropriate shock in the Comparison of Medical Therapy, Pacing, and Defibrillation in Heart Failure (COMPANION) Trial. Circulation 2006;114(25):2766–72.

23. Cleland JG, Daubert JC, Erdmann E, et al. Longer-term effects of cardiac resynchronization therapy on mortality in heart failure [the CArdiac REsynchronization-Heart Failure (CARE-HF) trial extension phase]. Eur Heart J 2006;27(16):1928–32.

24. Abraham WT, Fisher WG, Smith AL, et al. Cardiac resynchronization in chronic heart failure. N Engl J Med 2002;346(24):1845–53.

25. St John Sutton MG, Plappert T, Abraham WT, et al. Effect of cardiac resynchronization therapy on left ventricular size and function in chronic heart failure. Circulation 2003;107(15):1985–90.

26. Young JB, Abraham WT, Smith AL, et al. Combined cardiac resynchronization and implantable cardioversion defibrillation in advanced chronic heart failure: the MIRACLE ICD Trial. JAMA 2003;289(20):2685–94.

27. Cazeau S, Leclercq C, Lavergne T, et al. Effects of multisite biventricular pacing in patients with heart failure and intraventricular conduction delay. N Engl J Med 2001;344(12):873–80.

28. Leclercq C, Walker S, Linde C, et al. Comparative effects of permanent biventricular and right-univentricular pacing in heart failure patients with chronic atrial fibrillation. Eur Heart J 2002;23(22):1780–7.

29. Linde C, Leclercq C, Rex S, et al. Long-term benefits of biventricular pacing in congestive heart failure: results from the MUltisite STimulation in cardiomyopathy (MUSTIC) study. J Am Coll Cardiol 2002;40(1):111–8.

30. Auricchio A, Stellbrink C, Sack S, et al. Long-term clinical effect of hemodynamically optimized cardiac resynchronization therapy in patients with heart

failure and ventricular conduction delay. J Am Coll Cardiol 2002;39(12):2026–33.

31. Higgins SL, Hummel JD, Niazi IK, et al. Cardiac resynchronization therapy for the treatment of heart failure in patients with intraventricular conduction delay and malignant ventricular tachyarrhythmias. J Am Coll Cardiol 2003;42(8):1454–9.

32. Kindermann M, Hennen B, Jung J, et al. Biventricular versus conventional right ventricular stimulation for patients with standard pacing indication and left ventricular dysfunction: the Homburg Biventricular Pacing Evaluation (HOBIPACE). J Am Coll Cardiol 2006;47(10):1927–37.

33. Linde C, Abraham WT, Gold MR, et al. Randomized trial of cardiac resynchronization in mildly symptomatic heart failure patients and in asymptomatic patients with left ventricular dysfunction and previous heart failure symptoms. J Am Coll Cardiol 2008;52(23):1834–43.

34. Zipes DP, Camm AJ, Borggrefe M, et al. ACC/AHA/ESC 2006 guidelines for management of patients with ventricular arrhythmias and the prevention of sudden cardiac death—executive summary: a report of the American College of Cardiology/American Heart Association Task Force and the European Society of Cardiology Committee for Practice Guidelines (Writing Committee to Develop Guidelines for Management of Patients with Ventricular Arrhythmias and the Prevention of Sudden Cardiac Death): developed in Collaboration with the European Heart Rhythm Association and the Heart Rhythm Society. Eur Heart J 2006;27(17):2099–140.

35. Epstein AE, DiMarco JP, Ellenbogen KA, et al. ACC/AHA/HRS 2008 Guidelines for Device-Based Therapy of Cardiac Rhythm Abnormalities: a report of the American College of Cardiology/American Heart Association Task Force on Practice Guidelines (Writing Committee to Revise the ACC/AHA/NASPE 2002 Guideline Update for Implantation of Cardiac Pacemakers and Antiarrhythmia Devices): developed in collaboration with the American Association for Thoracic Surgery and Society of Thoracic Surgeons. Circulation 2008;117(21):e350–408.

36. Mark DB, Anstrom KJ, Sun JL, et al. Quality of life with defibrillator therapy or amiodarone in heart failure. N Engl J Med 2008;359(10):999–1008.

37. Theuns DA, Smith T, Hunink MG, et al. Effectiveness of prophylactic implantation of cardioverter-defibrillators without cardiac resynchronization therapy in patients with ischaemic or non-ischaemic heart disease: a systematic review and meta-analysis. Europace 2010;12(11):1564–70.

38. Hohnloser SH, Kuck KH, Dorian P, et al. Prophylactic use of an implantable cardioverter-defibrillator after acute myocardial infarction. N Engl J Med 2004;351(24):2481–8.

39. Steinbeck G, Andresen D, Seidl K, et al. Defibrillator implantation early after myocardial infarction. N Engl J Med 2009;361(15):1427–36.

40. Al-Khatib SM, Hellkamp A, Curtis J, et al. Non-evidence-based ICD implantations in the United States. JAMA 2011;305(1):43–9.

41. Dorian P, Hohnloser SH, Thorpe KE, et al. Mechanisms underlying the lack of effect of implantable cardioverter-defibrillator therapy on mortality in high-risk patients with recent myocardial infarction: insights from the defibrillation in acute myocardial infarction trial (DINAMIT). Circulation 2010;122(25):2645–52.

42. Sweeney MO. The contradiction of appropriate shocks in primary prevention ICDs: increasing and decreasing the risk of death. Circulation 2010;122(25):2638–41.

43. Knight BP. Implantable cardioverter-defibrillators: clinical trials of primary prevention of sudden cardiac death. UpToDate Online 18.3. 2009. Available at: http://www.uptodate.com. Accessed December 14, 2010.

44. Strickberger SA, Hummel JD, Bartlett TG, et al. Amiodarone versus implantable cardioverter-defibrillator: randomized trial in patients with nonischemic dilated cardiomyopathy and asymptomatic nonsustained ventricular tachycardia—AMIOVIRT. J Am Coll Cardiol 2003;41(10):1707–12.

45. Bigger JT Jr. Prophylactic use of implanted cardiac defibrillators in patients at high risk for ventricular arrhythmias after coronary-artery bypass graft surgery. Coronary Artery Bypass Graft (CABG) Patch Trial Investigators. N Engl J Med 1997;337(22):1569–75.

46. Bansch D, Antz M, Boczor S, et al. Primary prevention of sudden cardiac death in idiopathic dilated cardiomyopathy: the Cardiomyopathy Trial (CAT). Circulation 2002;105(12):1453–8.

47. Kadish A, Dyer A, Daubert JP, et al. Prophylactic defibrillator implantation in patients with nonischemic dilated cardiomyopathy. N Engl J Med 2004;350(21):2151–8.

48. Desai AS, Fang JC, Maisel WH, et al. Implantable defibrillators for the prevention of mortality in patients with nonischemic cardiomyopathy: a meta-analysis of randomized controlled trials. JAMA 2004;292(23):2874–9.

49. Causes of death in the Antiarrhythmics Versus Implantable Defibrillators (AVID) Trial. J Am Coll Cardiol 1999;34(5):1552–9.

50. Lee DS, Green LD, Liu PP, et al. Effectiveness of implantable defibrillators for preventing arrhythmic events and death: a meta-analysis. J Am Coll Cardiol 2003;41(9):1573–82.

51. Saba S, Atiga WL, Barrington W, et al. Selected patients listed for cardiac transplantation may benefit from defibrillator implantation regardless of

an established indication. J Heart Lung Transplant 2003;22(4):411–8.

52. Ghanbari H, Dalloul G, Hasan R, et al. Effectiveness of implantable cardioverter-defibrillators for the primary prevention of sudden cardiac death in women with advanced heart failure: a meta-analysis of randomized controlled trials. Arch Intern Med 2009;169(16):1500–6.

53. Peterson PN, Daugherty SL, Wang Y, et al. Gender differences in procedure-related adverse events in patients receiving implantable cardioverter-defibrillator therapy. Circulation 2009;119(8): 1078–84.

54. Santangeli P, Di Biase L, Dello Russo A, et al. Meta-analysis: age and effectiveness of prophylactic implantable cardioverter-defibrillators. Ann Intern Med 2010;153(9):592–9.

55. Hernandez AF, Fonarow GC, Hammill BG, et al. Clinical effectiveness of implantable cardioverter-defibrillators among Medicare beneficiaries with heart failure. Circ Heart Fail 2010;3(1):7–13.

56. Chan PS, Nallamothu BK, Spertus JA, et al. Impact of age and medical comorbidity on the effectiveness of implantable cardioverter-defibrillators for primary prevention. Circ Cardiovasc Qual Outcomes 2009; 2(1):16–24.

57. Epstein AE, Kay GN, Plumb VJ, et al. Implantable cardioverter-defibrillator prescription in the elderly. Heart Rhythm 2009;6(8):1136–43.

58. Goldenberg I, Moss AJ, McNitt S, et al. Relations among renal function, risk of sudden cardiac death, and benefit of the implanted cardiac defibrillator in patients with ischemic left ventricular dysfunction. Am J Cardiol 2006;98(4):485–90.

59. Aggarwal A, Wang Y, Rumsfeld JS, et al. Clinical characteristics and in-hospital outcome of patients with end-stage renal disease on dialysis referred for implantable cardioverter-defibrillator implantation. Heart Rhythm 2009;6(11):1565–71.

60. Freeman JV, Wang Y, Curtis JP, et al. The relation between hospital procedure volume and complications of cardioverter-defibrillator implantation from the implantable cardioverter-defibrillator registry. J Am Coll Cardiol 2010;56(14):1133–9.

61. Kuhlkamp V, Dornberger V, Mewis C, et al. Clinical experience with the new detection algorithms for atrial fibrillation of a defibrillator with dual chamber sensing and pacing. J Cardiovasc Electrophysiol 1999;10(7):905–15.

62. Deisenhofer I, Kolb C, Ndrepepa G, et al. Do current dual chamber cardioverter defibrillators have advantages over conventional single chamber cardioverter defibrillators in reducing inappropriate therapies? A randomized, prospective study. J Cardiovasc Electrophysiol 2001;12(2):134–42.

63. Theuns DA, Klootwijk AP, Goedhart DM, et al. Prevention of inappropriate therapy in implantable cardioverter-defibrillators: results of a prospective, randomized study of tachyarrhythmia detection algorithms. J Am Coll Cardiol 2004;44(12):2362–7.

64. Dorian P, Philippon F, Thibault B, et al. Randomized controlled study of detection enhancements versus rate-only detection to prevent inappropriate therapy in a dual-chamber implantable cardioverter-defibrillator. Heart Rhythm 2004; 1(5):540–7.

65. Bansch D, Steffgen F, Gronefeld G, et al. The 1+1 trial: a prospective trial of a dual- versus a single-chamber implantable defibrillator in patients with slow ventricular tachycardias. Circulation 2004; 110(9):1022–9.

66. Friedman PA, McClelland RL, Bamlet WR, et al. Dual-chamber versus single-chamber detection enhancements for implantable defibrillator rhythm diagnosis: the detect supraventricular tachycardia study. Circulation 2006;113(25):2871–9.

67. Theuns DA, Rivero-Ayerza M, Boersma E, et al. Prevention of inappropriate therapy in implantable defibrillators: a meta-analysis of clinical trials comparing single-chamber and dual-chamber arrhythmia discrimination algorithms. Int J Cardiol 2008;125(3):352–7.

68. Curtis JP, Luebbert JJ, Wang Y, et al. Association of physician certification and outcomes among patients receiving an implantable cardioverter-defibrillator. JAMA 2009;301(16):1661–70.

69. Lam SK, Owen A. Combined resynchronisation and implantable defibrillator therapy in left ventricular dysfunction: Bayesian network meta-analysis of randomised controlled trials. BMJ 2007; 335(7626):925.

70. Anand IS, Carson P, Galle E, et al. Cardiac resynchronization therapy reduces the risk of hospitalizations in patients with advanced heart failure: results from the Comparison of Medical Therapy, Pacing and Defibrillation in Heart Failure (COMPANION) trial. Circulation 2009;119(7): 969–77.

71. McAlister FA, Ezekowitz J, Hooton N, et al. Cardiac resynchronization therapy for patients with left ventricular systolic dysfunction: a systematic review. JAMA 2007;297(22):2502–14.

72. Fein AS, Wang Y, Curtis JP, et al. Prevalence and predictors of off-label use of cardiac resynchronization therapy in patients enrolled in the National Cardiovascular Data Registry Implantable Cardiac-Defibrillator Registry. J Am Coll Cardiol 2010; 56(10):766–73.

73. Lindenfeld J, Feldman AM, Saxon L, et al. Effects of cardiac resynchronization therapy with or without a defibrillator on survival and hospitalizations in patients with New York Heart Association class IV heart failure. Circulation 2007;115(2): 204–12.

74. Germany RE, Ripley TL. Controversies in cardiac resynchronization therapy: do sex differences in response exist? Curr Heart Fail Rep 2011;8(1):59–64.

75. Bilchick KC, Kamath S, DiMarco JP, et al. Bundle-branch block morphology and other predictors of outcome after cardiac resynchronization therapy in Medicare patients. Circulation 2010;122(20): 2022–30.

76. Jessup M, Abraham WT, Casey DE, et al. 2009 focused update: ACCF/AHA Guidelines for the Diagnosis and Management of Heart Failure in Adults: a report of the American College of Cardiology Foundation/American Heart Association Task Force on Practice Guidelines: developed in collaboration with the International Society for Heart and Lung Transplantation. Circulation 2009;119(14):1977–2016.

Comparative Effectiveness Research in Heart Failure Therapies
Women, Elderly Patients, and Patients with Kidney Disease

Rashmee U. Shah, MD, MS[a],*, Tara I. Chang, MD, MS[b],
Gregg C. Fonarow, MD[c]

KEYWORDS

- Heart failure • Comparative effectiveness • Women • Elderly • Chronic renal insufficiency

KEY POINTS

- Comparative effectiveness research is a key component in improving heart failure (HF) management.
- Many of the patients in clinical practice are dissimilar to the patients in randomized controlled trials, so alternative sources of information must guide treatment.
- There is reasonable evidence to support the use of most HF therapeutics in women but less evidence to support use in older patients and patients with kidney disease.

No two patients have an identical form of the disease and it was desired to eliminate as many of the obvious variations as possible. This planning is a fundamental feature of the successful trial. To start out upon a trial with all and sundry included, and with the hope that the results can be sorted out statistically in the end is to court disaster.
— Sir A.B. Hill, 1951[1]

INTRODUCTION

The incidence and prevalence of heart failure (HF) has increased during recent decades as a result of an aging population and improvements in treatment and survival of cardiovascular disease. Morbidity and mortality for HF are substantial, with more than 1.1 million hospital discharges in 2006 and almost 3.5 million outpatient visits in 2007. Estimated direct and indirect costs in 2010 amount to almost $40 billion.[2]

Randomized controlled trials (RCTs) have identified effective HF treatments, but the patients included in these trials often represent a select subgroup of all patients with HF. RCT participants are often male, young, and with fewer and less severe comorbid conditions. Conversely, HF patients in daily practice are often old, female,

Funding: Drs Shah and Chang are supported by a grant from the American Heart Association Pharmaceutical Round Table. Dr Shah is supported in part by the Stanford NIH/NCRR CTSA grant KL2 RR025743. Dr Fonarow is supported by the Ahmanson-UCLA Foundation (Los Angeles, CA) and holds the Eliot Corday Chair of Cardiovascular Medicine.
Conflicts of interest: None.
[a] Cedars-Sinai Medical Center, Department of Cardiology, 8700 Beverly Blvd Room 5536B, CA 90048, USA;
[b] Department of Medicine, Stanford University, 780 Welch Road, Suite 106, Palo Alto, CA 94304, USA;
[c] Department of Medicine, University of California Los Angeles, 10833 LeConte Avenue, Los Angeles, CA 90095, USA
* Corresponding author.
E-mail address: rashmee.shah@cshs.org

heartfailure.theclinics.com

and with extensive comorbid conditions.[3,4] Thus, one is left with the dilemma described in the quote above: How can one determine effective treatments for HF populations that are underrepresented in RCTs?

The recently coined term "comparative effectiveness research" (CER) describes a field that aims to fill in the gaps in the evidence base. CER is defined, in part, as research that provides "direct comparison of effective interventions and their study in patients who are typical of day-to-day clinical care.[5]" This article discusses methodological considerations in CER followed by a review of existing CER for pharmacologic management in HF, focusing on 3 special patient populations with HF: women, older patients, and patients with kidney disease.

METHODOLOGICAL CONSIDERATIONS FOR CER

Conventional RCTs commonly enroll the minimum number of patients required to establish efficacy and are generally not well powered to evaluate efficacy in clinically relevant subgroups. This methodology poses a significant challenge when providing treatment recommendations or formulating guidelines that can be generalized to underrepresented patient populations.

RCT design could include certain methodological approaches to minimize bias among subgroups and allow for CER. One option is to recruit a large sample of patients using minimally restrictive inclusion and exclusion criteria—the "large sample trial." In this way, the population enrolled more closely resembles the target population with the disease.

Analyses of trial data can assess treatment effect similarities across patient subgroups, with the groups of interest specified a priori. The first step is to examine outcomes in each subgroup, typically displayed in a forest diagram; the next is to test for subgroup by treatment interaction in a regression model. If a significant interaction emerges, then stratified subgroup analysis is justified. Investigators and readers should be cautious about multiplicity in subgroup analysis: the more the number of hypotheses that are tested, the more likely that the results are significant due to of chance alone. For example, at a significance of alpha = 0.05, 10 subgroup comparisons yield a 40% probability that one of the conclusions is due to chance alone; 5 subgroup comparisons yield a 23% probability that one of the conclusions is due to chance alone.[1,6]

With the preponderance of evidence to support certain HF therapies, additional RCTs to address special populations are unlikely. CER with observational, nonrandomized data may be useful in examining outcomes in subgroups that are underrepresented in RCTs. However, the treatment groups may not be comparable because the choice to treat is often related to patient characteristics, which are also related to the outcome. Several quasiexperimental study designs can address this limitation, and interested readers are referred to the references for more information about these advanced methods.[7–9]

WOMEN

Women represent almost 60% of incident HF cases and HF hospitalizations but only 20%–30% of clinical trial participants.[3] Disease characteristics differ between the sexes: antecedent hypertension and preserved ejection fraction are more prevalent among women, whereas antecedent coronary artery disease is less prevalent among women compared with men with HF.[10,11] Because there is biological potential for women to respond differently to various HF therapies compared with men, establishing efficacy and effectiveness of each specific HF therapy in women is important.

Beta-Blockers

Beta-blockers have the most evidence supporting their use in women with HF and reduced left ventricular ejection fraction (LVEF) (**Table 1**). Three major beta-blocker RCTs included subgroup or post hoc analysis to examine sex-specific treatment effect. A post hoc analysis of the Metoprolol CR/XL Randomized Intervention Trial in Congestive Heart Failure (MERIT-HF) showed a nonsignificant sex by treatment interaction ($P = .14$).[12,13] In the stratified analysis, metoprolol treatment yielded a 21% decrease in the combined end point of hospitalizations and death in women ($P = .044$), compared with an 18% decrease in men ($P = .001$). Stratified analyses from 2 carvedilol RCTs, as well as the results of pooled trials and meta-analysis of beta-blocker trials, also support the benefits of beta-blocker use in women with HF and reduced LVEF.[14–16]

Observational studies also suggest that beta-blockers are clinically effective in both women and men with HF. One such study used a large, Canadian discharge database and examined outcomes after HF hospitalization according to beta-blocker prescription. In the sex-stratified analysis, beta-blockers conferred similar survival benefits in men and women; no sex by treatment interaction was found.[17] Another study of patients with HF discharged with beta-blocker therapy showed that patients with reduced LVEF had a significantly lower risk-adjusted mortality. In contrast, both men and

Table 1
Characteristics of selected beta-blocker trials with mortality benefit

Study	Inclusion Criteria	Intervention	Mean Age (Years)	Percentage of Women (n/Total)	CKD Exclusion	Subgroup Analysis
US Carvedilol Heart Failure Study[14]	Symptomatic HF and EF ≤35%	Carvedilol vs placebo	58.0	23 (256/1094)	Clinically important renal disease	Yes
Carvedilol Prospective Randomized Cumulative Survival Study[15]	NYHA class IV HF and EF ≤25%	Carvedilol vs placebo	63.3	21 (470/2289)	Creatinine ≥2.8 mg/dL	Yes
Metoprolol CR/XL Randomized Intervention Trial in Congestive Heart Failure[12,67]	NYHA class II–IV HF and EF ≤40%	Metoprolol succinate vs placebo	63.8	23 (898/3991)	None	Yes
Cardiac Insufficiency Bisoprolol Study II[49]	NYHA class III–IV HF and EF ≤35%	Bisoprolol vs placebo	61.0	19 (515/2647)	Creatinine ≥3.4 mg/dL	No[a]
Study of the Effects of Nebivolol Intervention on Outcomes and Rehospitalization in Seniors with Heart Failure[34,68]	Age ≥70 y and EF ≤35% or HF hospitalization within the previous 12 mo	Nebivolol vs placebo	76.1	37 (785/2128)	Creatinine ≥2.8 mg/dL	Yes
Carvedilol or Metoprolol European Trial[69,70]		Carvedilol vs metoprolol tartrate	62.0	20 (612/3029)	Serious systemic disease with reduced life expectancy	Yes

Abbreviations: EF, ejection fraction; NYHA, New York Heart Association.
[a] Included subgroup analysis, but not related to age, sex, or kidney function.

women with preserved LVEF derived no benefit from beta-blocker therapy.[18]

Angiotensin-Converting Enzyme Inhibitors and Angiotensin II Receptor Blockers

Several RCTs have demonstrated that angiotensin-converting enzyme (ACE) inhibitor treatment in patients with HF and reduced LVEF reduces mortality (**Table 2**), and a meta-analysis demonstrated similar treatment effects in both men and women. The meta-analysis included 7 trials and 2898 women; the investigators found a relative risk (RR) of 0.92 (95% confidence interval [CI], 0.81–1.04) for mortality in treated women, compared with 0.82 (95% CI, 0.74–0.90) in men. Although the confidence interval for the treatment effect in women crosses 1, the sex-specific estimates were statistically similar.[16] Observational studies also support the use of ACE inhibitors in women with HF and reduced LVEF.[19]

The Candesartan in Heart failure Assessment of Reduction in Mortality (CHARM-Overall) trial included 2400 women and provided a sex by treatment interaction analysis. The primary outcome, time to cardiovascular death or HF admission, was reduced by 18% in the treatment arm, with an insignificant sex by treatment interaction term ($P = .87$).[20]

Aldosterone Receptor Antagonists

Aldosterone receptor antagonists were tested in 3 large RCTs in patients with reduced LVEF (**Table 3**). The Randomized Aldactone Evaluation Study (RALES) showed a significant reduction in mortality in the treatment arm, with similar effects in men and women.[21] Results from the Eplerenone Post-Acute Myocardial Infarction Efficacy and Survival Study (EPHESUS) showed a 15% reduction in all-cause mortality; in the sex-stratified analysis, the mortality reduction was significant for women but not for men. However, the sex by treatment interaction term was insignificant ($P = .44$), suggesting similar effects in men and women.[22]

More recently, the Eplerenone in Mild Patients Hospitalization and Survival Study in Heart Failure (EMPHASIS-HF) study provided further support for aldosterone receptor antagonists in women. In this RCT in mild HF with reduced LVEF, eplerenone significantly reduced all-cause mortality by 24% (adjusted hazard ratio [HR], 0.76; 95% CI, 0.62–0.93) and the primary end point of death from cardiovascular cause or HF hospitalization by 27% (adjusted HR, 0.63; 95% CI, 0.54–0.74). The sex by treatment interaction term was nonsignificant, and the sex-stratified analysis

revealed significant reduction in the primary end point for both men and women treated with eplerenone.[23]

Digoxin

Among the HF therapies, the Digoxin Investigators Group (DIG) trial results received much publicity for sex-specific treatment effects. The original investigation found that digoxin had a significant effect on HF hospitalization but did not alter mortality.[24] A subsequent post hoc analysis revealed more deaths among women in the treatment arm, 33.1% versus 28.9%, and a significant sex by treatment interaction term ($P = .014$),[25] suggesting that there may be increased drug toxicity in women. Further investigations of the DIG trial showed that sex-specific treatment effects disappeared at lower serum digoxin levels.[26] The findings of the DIG trial have not been confirmed in other studies.

Summary

Evaluation from RCTs and CER thus far suggests that most HF therapies have similar treatment effects in men and women, with the possible exception of digoxin. However, the studies described earlier have limitations. None were designed to specifically test sex by treatment interactions. Furthermore, HF with preserved LVEF is more common among women, but almost all RCTs include only patients with reduced LVEF and there are few observational studies of treatment in patients with preserved LVEF. As a result, there is no reliable evidence on which to base treatment of many women with HF seen in daily clinical practice. Several RCTs are underway to test various therapies in patients with HF and preserved LVEF and should shed light on treatment of women.[27–29]

ELDERLY PATIENTS

The prevalence of HF increases from 2% to 3% at age 65 years to more than 80% in persons older than 80 years. HF is also the most common reason for hospitalization in elderly patients. The average age of HF onset is more than 75 years; this figure approaches 80 years in the Medicare population.[30,31] Yet, the mean age of RCT participants is 61 years and many older patients with HF do not meet enrollment criteria.[3,4] Comorbid conditions account for many of the RCT exclusions, although some trials exclude patients based on age alone. Older patients may metabolize medications differently compared with younger patients and may experience higher risk of adverse

Table 2
Characteristics of selected angiotensin-converting enzyme inhibitor trials with mortality benefit

Study	Inclusion Criteria	Intervention	Mean Age (Years)	Percentage of Women (n/Total)	CKD Exclusion	Subgroup Analysis
Cooperative North Scandinavian Enalapril Survival Study[54]	NYHA Class IV HF and clinical signs/symptoms of HF	Enalapril vs placebo	70.5	23 (59/253)	Creatinine ≥3.4 mg/dL	No
Studies of Left Ventricular Dysfunction—Treatment[53]	HF and EF ≤35%	Enalapril vs placebo	60.8	20 (505/2569)	Creatinine ≥2.0 mg/dL	No[a]
Studies of Left Ventricular Dysfunction—Prevention[61]	EF ≤35% and no treatment of HF (diuretics, digoxin, vasodilators)	Enalapril vs placebo	59.1	7 (294/4228)	Creatinine ≥2.0 mg/dL or dialysis	No[a]
Acute Infarction Ramipril Efficacy Study[71,72]	AMI and signs/symptoms of HF	Ramipril vs placebo	65.0	26 (525/1986)	Recognized contraindications to ACE-I therapy	Yes
Survival of Myocardial Infarction Long-Term Evaluation Study[73]	Anterior wall myocardial infarction	Zofenopril vs placebo	64.1	27 (428/1556)	Creatinine ≥2.5 mg/dL	Yes
Trandolapril Cardiac Evaluation Study[74]	Acute myocardial infarction and EF ≤35%	Trandolapril vs placebo	67.5	28 (498/1749)	Creatinine ≥2.3 mg/dL	Yes
Survival and Ventricular Enlargement Trial[75]	AMI and EF ≤40%	Captopril vs placebo	59.4	18 (390/2231)	Creatinine ≥2.5 mg/dL	No

Abbreviations: EF, ejection fraction; NYHA, New York Heart Association.
a Included subgroup analysis, but not related to age, sex, or kidney function.

Table 3
Characteristics of selected aldosterone antagonist trials with mortality benefit

Study	Inclusion Criteria	Intervention	Mean Age (Years)	Percentage of Women (n/Total)	CKD Exclusion	Subgroup Analysis
The Randomized Aldactone Evaluation Study[21]	NYHA Class II or IV HF and EF ≤35%	Spironolactone vs placebo	65.0	27 (446/1663)	Creatinine ≥2.5 mg/dL	Yes
Eplerenone Post-Acute Myocardial Infarction Efficacy and Survival Study[22]	Acute myocardial infarction and EF ≤40%	Eplerenone vs placebo	64.0	29 (1918/6632)	Creatinine ≥2.5 mg/dL	Yes
Eplerenone in Mild Patients Hospitalization and Survival Study in Heart Failure[23]	NYHA Class II HF, age ≥55 y, EF ≤35%	Eplerenone vs placebo	68.6	22 (610/2737)	eGFR ≤30 mL/min/1.73 m^2	Yes

Abbreviations: EF, ejection fraction; NYHA, New York Heart Association.

effects attributable to treatment. Thus, establishing effectiveness and safety of each specific HF therapy in the older patient population with HF is important.

Beta-Blockers

Stratified analyses of beta-blocker RCTs by age are limited because of small sample sizes, particularly for the oldest patients (see **Table 1**). In the US Carvedilol Heart Failure Study, the investigators divided the cohort into older and younger than 59 years old and found mortality benefit in both age groups.[14] In the second carvedilol RCT, COPERNICUS, the investigators stratified at age 65 years and found similar treatment effects in older and younger groups.[15] A post hoc analysis of MERIT-HF studied trial participants aged 65 years and older and found a 37% reduction in all-cause mortality (RR, 0.63; 95% CI, 0.48–0.83) among patients treated with metoprolol succinate, with a trend toward benefit in patients aged 75 years and older (RR, 0.71; 95% CI, 0.42–1.19). Older patients treated with metoprolol did not have an increased rate of adverse events (such as bronchospasm, depression, and dizziness) that resulted in therapy discontinuation.[32]

Two investigations have focused exclusively on older patients with HF, including the Carvedilol Open Assessment II (COLA II) study and the Study of the Effects of Nebivolol Intervention on Outcomes and Rehospitalization in Seniors with Heart Failure (SENIORS). In the COLA II study, more than 1000 patients with HF aged 70 years and older were followed up after administering carvedilol; more than 80% of the recipients continued the medication for 3 or more months, suggesting that side-effect concerns should not limit beta-blocker prescription to elderly patients with HF.[33] SENIORS was an RCT of nebivolol, including patients with HF aged 70 years and older with reduced LVEF. The investigators found a significant reduction in the combined outcome of all-cause mortality and cardiovascular hospitalization in the nebivolol arm (HR, 0.86; 95% CI, 0.74–0.99) but no significant effect on all-cause mortality (HR, 0.88; 95% CI, 0.71–1.08).[34]

The Organized Program to Initiate Lifesaving Treatment in Hospitalized Patients with Heart Failure (OPTIMIZE-HF) study provides important observational data in support of beta-blocker treatment in the elderly. This registry included patients with a median age of approximately 80 years, with one-fourth of patients older than 85 years; more than half the patients had preserved LVEF. Among patients with reduced LVEF, beta-

blocker therapy yielded a 23% mortality reduction and the age by treatment interaction term was nonsignificant (P = .87). Beta-blocker therapy did not improve outcomes in patients with preserved LVEF.[18]

ACE Inhibitors and Angiotensin II Receptor Blockers

Flather and colleagues[35] performed a meta-analysis of 5 ACE inhibitor trials (see **Table 2**) and included a subgroup analysis by age. They found a significant 20% reduction in all-cause mortality among those treated with ACE inhibitors and a nonsignificant age by treatment interaction term (P = .47). In the subgroup analysis, mortality was significantly reduced among patients aged 65 to 75 years. For patients older than 75 years, mortality was reduced by 5%, although the confidence interval crossed 1, probably because of the small sample size.[35] Although the age by treatment interaction term was nonsignificant, a firm conclusion cannot be drawn about patients older than 75 years.

Observational studies also support the use of ACE inhibitors in older patients with reduced LVEF. A publication from the National Heart Care Project, a Center for Medicare and Medicaid Services initiative, reported that ACE inhibitor use among Medicare beneficiaries resulted in a 14% relative reduction in 1-year mortality risk (RR, 0.86; 95% CI, 0.82–0.90). Furthermore, this study stratified the cohort according to age and found that the oldest old (age 85 years and older) had an apparent mortality benefit with ACE inhibitors or angiotensin II receptor blockers (ARBs).[36]

The CHARM-Overall trial, which found a mortality benefit for patients with HF treated with candesartan, also performed a subgroup analysis according to age. The study reported a significant mortality benefit for patients aged 65 to 75 years and older than 75 years; the age by treatment interaction term was nonsignificant (P = .26).[20]

Aldosterone Receptor Antagonists

Both RALES and EPHESUS examined outcomes by age (see **Table 3**). RALES found a significant mortality reduction for patients aged 67 years and older treated with spironoalctone.[21] EPHESUS reported a nonsignificant age by treatment interaction (P = .23) for patients treated with eplerenone.[22] EMPAHSIS-HF also reported an age-stratified analysis, which showed no evidence of treatment heterogeneity between younger and older participants.[23]

Digoxin

The original DIG trial publication did not report age-stratified results, so one must rely on post hoc analysis to infer treatment effects in elderly patients with HF. Ahmed and colleagues[26] examined outcomes according to serum digoxin levels and found that patients with levels 0.5 to 0.9 ng/dL experienced a 23% reduction in all-cause mortality. In the age-stratified analysis, the treatment effect was similar in patients aged 70 years and older. In addition, age was a significant predictor of higher drug levels, suggesting that with careful dosing and close monitoring, older patients may benefit from digoxin.

Summary

Evidence regarding the effectiveness and safety of HF treatment among older patients is limited, mainly because of patient exclusions from RCTs. Although age-stratified analyses suggest that HF therapies are effective for older patients, the very old (ie, age 80 years and older) are rarely included in RCTs. In addition, comorbid conditions are the norm among older patients seen in daily practice, a feature that is not represented in RCT participants.[37] Thus, it is difficult to draw firm conclusions from RCTs about how to treat older patients with HF. Observational data can provide some insight, but accounting for confounders in a nonrandomized design is difficult.

CER for older patients with HF should focus on safety, in addition to mortality and morbidity outcomes, because older patients are more prone to adverse events and side effects.[38,39] The importance of safety outcomes was highlighted in an investigation following the publication of RALES, which illustrated increased hyperkalemia and hyperkalemia-associated deaths among an HF cohort aged 65 years and older.[40] Although it is difficult to address safety outcomes because of the low occurrence of adverse events, these investigations are particularly important in CER pertaining to older patients, who are more likely to have HF with preserved LVEF. Identifying therapies that are safe and effective in patients with preserved LVEF will be particularly applicable to the cohort of older patients with HF.

KIDNEY DISEASE

More than two-thirds of patients with HF also have kidney disease.[41–43] Kidney disease severity has been shown to predict mortality in patients with HF and has consistently been shown to be an independent risk factor for adverse cardiovascular events and mortality in broader populations.[43–46] Medications such as renin-angiotension-aldosterone system (RAAS) inhibitors and beta-blockers reduce HF mortality and morbidity in the general population with HF, but little is known about their treatment effectiveness and safety in patients with HF and kidney disease. Most HF RCTs have excluded patients with elevated serum creatinine concentrations and/or reduced estimated glomerular filtration rates (eGFR).

Beta-Blockers

Post hoc analyses of beta-blocker RCTs provide evidence to support the use of beta-blockers in patients with HF and mild to moderate kidney disease (see **Table 1**). MERIT-HF reported a 19% (95% CI, 10%–27%) lower risk in the primary end point of all-cause mortality or first hospitalization.[47] A subsequent secondary analysis of MERIT-HF data showed similar benefit in all-cause mortality across categories of eGFR (P for interaction = .095).[48] However, very few patients had an eGFR of less than 45 mL/min/1.73 m^2, given the exclusion criteria of the original trial.

The Cardiac Insufficiency Bisoprolol Study II (CIBIS-II) reported a 34% (95% CI, 19%–56%) lower risk of all-cause mortality in the beta-blocker group.[49] A subsequent secondary analysis showed that approximately one-third of patients in the bisoprolol and placebo groups had an estimated creatinine clearance of less than 30 mL/min and found similar reductions in all-cause mortality after stratifying by creatinine clearance.[50] The SENIORS trial found similar benefits of nebivolol, but included only patients with mildly reduced kidney function.[34,51]

To date, there has been only 1 RCT of beta-blockers in patients with end-stage renal disease (ESRD) on hemodialysis with HF.[52] In that study, all patients had an LVEF of less than 35% and symptomatic HF. At 2 years, the group receiving carvedilol demonstrated a 49% (95% CI, 18%–68%) lower risk of all-cause mortality compared with patients receiving placebo and also experienced fewer HF hospitalizations than the placebo group.

Because of the consistent benefit seen across categories of kidney function in several trials, as well as the support from large-scale observational studies,[18,42] beta-blockers seem to be effective in patients with HF with various degrees of kidney disease.

ACE Inhibitors

Two major RCTs showing benefit of ACE inhibitors in reducing mortality in symptomatic patients with HF, the Studies of Left Ventricular Dysfunction (SOLVD)[53] and Cooperative North Scandinavian

Enalapril Survival Study (CONSENSUS)[54] trials, included significant proportions of patients with kidney disease (see **Table 2**). Patients in the SOLVD-Treatment trial randomized to receive enalapril had a 16% (95% CI, 5%–26%) lower risk of all-cause mortality compared with patients randomized to placebo. Although the SOLVD-Treatment trial excluded patients with serum creatinine concentrations greater than 2.5 mg/dL, approximately 36% of patients had an eGFR less than 60 mL/min.[44] Similarly, CONSENSUS showed reduced 6-month mortality rates in patients with severe HF treated with enalapril and had a liberal creatinine cutoff, allowing serum creatinine concentrations up to 3.4 mg/dL. Although neither trial formally assessed kidney disease in subgroup analyses, these data, along with results from observational studies,[42] provide support for the use of ACE inhibitors in patients with mild kidney disease and HF.

Angiotensin Receptor Blockers

ARBs are recommended for the treatment of HF among patients who cannot tolerate ACE inhibitors. Although some ARB RCTs included subgroup analyses for patients with kidney disease, most of these trials excluded patients with more advanced kidney disease. For example, a post hoc analysis of CHARM-Overall showed that candesartan was equally effective in the reduction in the primary end point in patients with a serum creatinine concentration of 2.0 mg/dL or greater versus less than 2.0 mg/dL (P for interaction = .63).[20] However, CHARM-Overall excluded patients with serum creatinine concentrations of 3.0 mg/dL or more.

The Heart failure Endpoint evaluation of Angiotensin II Antagonist Losartan (HEAAL) study is one of the few clinical trials that examined kidney disease as a prespecified subgroup.[55] In this trial comparing losartan 150 mg daily with losartan 50 mg daily, the higher dose of losartan was associated with a 10% (95% CI, 1%–18%) lower risk of death or HF hospitalization. These results did not differ by category of eGFR (P = .11 for interaction). However, as with CHARM, HEAAL excluded patients with a serum creatinine concentration greater than 2.5 mg/dL. Therefore, although ARBs seem to be effective for the treatment of patients with HF and mild kidney disease, there are no data regarding patients with HF and more severe kidney disease.

Aldosterone Antagonists

Aldosterone antagonists reduce mortality in the general population with HF and may be equally effective in patients with mild kidney disease (see **Table 3**). RALES demonstrated a 30% lower mortality rate in patients with severe HF randomized to receive spironolactone or placebo.[21] Kidney disease was a prespecified subgroup, and a similar benefit of spironolactone was seen in patients with a baseline serum creatinine concentration more than and less than 1.2 mg/dL. Improved mortality and morbidity in patients with HF and kidney disease has also been seen with eplerenone. Both EPHESUS and EMPHASIS-HF examined kidney disease as a prespecified subgroup and demonstrated similar benefits of eplerenone in patients with reduced kidney function as with higher kidney function.[22,23] However, as with RALES, EPHESUS excluded patients with serum creatinine concentrations greater than 2.5 mg/dL and EMPHASIS-HF excluded patients with eGFR less than 30 mL/min/1.73 m^2, so the effect of eplerenone among patients with more severe kidney disease is unknown.

RAAS Inhibitors in Patients with ESRD on Dialysis

There have been no RCTs to date of ACE inhibitors in patients with ESRD on dialysis and HF, and patients on dialysis have been excluded from RCTs of ACE inhibitors in the general population with HF. However, a study examined the addition of the ARB telmisartan to ACE inhibitors in patients on hemodialysis with symptomatic left HF.[52] In this 3-year study, patients receiving telmisartan experienced a 49% (95% CI, 39%–62%) lower risk of all-cause mortality, as well as lower risks of cardiovascular mortality and HF hospitalization. The remarkably large risk reduction is consistent with 2 previous studies of ARB monotherapy in patients on hemodialysis (but without HF),[56,57] but the possibility of false-positive results remains, because of the small sample sizes and the lack of significant benefit of ARBs added to ACE inhibitors on all-cause mortality seen in 2 large RCTs in the general population with HF.[58,59]

Safety of RAAS Inhibitors in Kidney Disease

ACE inhibitors decrease glomerular filtration pressure by dilating the efferent arteriolar in the glomerulus, which would be expected to increase serum creatinine concentration, particularly in patients with underlying kidney disease. A recent consensus statement from the National Kidney Foundation states that an increase in serum creatinine concentration is not of concern unless it exceeds 30% to 50% or does not stabilize by about 4 weeks after the initiation of the ACE inhibitor.[60] In SOLVD, a significantly larger proportion of patients treated with enalapril had an increase in serum creatinine levels to greater than 2.0 mg/dL compared with placebo (10.7% vs 7.7%, $P<.01$).[53] Similarly, in CONSENSUS, patients treated with enalapril had an increase in serum creatinine levels by 10% to 15% in the first 2 to 3 weeks of treatment, with a mean increase in serum creatinine levels of 14% at 24 weeks; no significant increase in the mean serum creatinine level was seen in the placebo group.[54] However, the rates of medication discontinuation due to increased serum creatinine levels were similar between the 2 groups.[53,54,61] Thirteen patients in CONSENSUS experienced a doubling of serum creatinine levels, most often associated with hypotension or intercurrent illnesses, which reversed on withdrawal of the ACE inhibitor, diuretic, or both.[62]

Hyperkalemia may also result after ACE inhibitor initiation in patients with HF and kidney disease. In SOLVD-Treatment, 6.4% of patients in the enalapril group had an increase in the serum potassium concentration to greater than 5.5 mmol/L, compared with 2.2% in the placebo group ($P<.01$). However, the clinical significance of the hyperkalemia in SOLVD-Treatment is unclear, as the number of patients who had to discontinue the ACE inhibitor as a result of hyperkalemia was not reported. A review of 6 clinical trials of ACE inhibitors in patients with moderate to advanced kidney disease, but without HF, found that only 2.0% of patients developed increases in serum potassium concentrations greater than 5.6 mmol/L and only 0.8% required termination of the ACE inhibitor as a result of hyperkalemia.[16] Because none of the trials included patients with systolic HF, the safety of ACE inhibitors in patients with concomitant kidney disease and HF cannot be assessed.

ARBs may also increase serum creatinine and potassium concentrations, as seen in CHARM-Alternative[63] and the Effect of Losartan in the Elderly (ELITE) trials. In the ELITE trial, which randomized patients to receive losartan or captopril, 10.5% of patients in both groups reached the primary end point of renal dysfunction, defined as an increase in the serum creatinine level by 0.3 mg/dL or more.[64] In patients with ESRD on dialysis, treatment with ARBs did not result in a greater incidence of hyperkalemia compared with placebo.[52,56,57]

Hyperkalemia is also a major concern when treating patients with HF and kidney disease with aldosterone antagonists. The incidence of serious hyperkalemia was remarkably low in RALES (2%),[21] whereas in EPHESUS, the rate of serious hyperkalemia was 10.1% in patients with a baseline creatinine clearance of less than 50 mL/min.[22] Moreover, aldosterone antagonists in a real-world setting may have higher adverse event rates. For example, a study conducted in Canada found a nearly threefold increase in hyperkalemia-associated hospitalizations and hyperkalemia-associated deaths after the publication of RALES.[40] Conversely, a study conducted in Scotland did not find an increase in hyperkalemia-associated adverse events.[65] In EPHESUS, the rate of serious hyperkalemia was 10.1% higher in patients with a baseline creatinine clearance of less than 50 mL/min.[22] Current guidelines provide recommendations for minimizing the risk of hyperkalemia in patients treated with aldosterone antagonists, including avoidance of concomitant use of nonsteroidal antiinflammatory drugs, discontinuation of potassium supplementation, smaller initial doses of aldosterone antagonists, and close monitoring of serum potassium and creatinine concentrations, especially in patients taking higher doses of ACE inhibitors. Aldosterone antagonists are not recommended in patients with creatinine clearances less than 30 mL/min or baseline serum potassium concentration greater than 5 meq/L.[66]

In summary, adverse effects such as increases in serum creatinine levels and hyperkalemia were uncommon and often reversible in the setting of a carefully monitored RCT but may be more common in the real-world clinical practice. Serum creatinine and potassium concentrations must be closely monitored when using RAAS inhibitors, especially in patients with more advanced kidney disease who are not yet on dialysis.

Digoxin

The original DIG trial excluded patients with a serum creatinine concentration greater than 3.0 mg/dL, and few patients had advanced kidney disease: 54% of the cohort had an eGFR greater than 60 mL/min/1.73 m^2, 43% had an eGFR of 30 to 60 mL/min/1.73 m^2, and only 3% had an eGFR less than 30 mL/min/1.73 m^2.[24] In a post hoc analysis, no benefit (and no increased risk) of digoxin on all-cause mortality or on the combined end point of death or HF hospitalization was seen across levels of kidney function (P for interaction = .19 and .54, respectively).[46]

Summary

At present, there is limited CER regarding the appropriate treatment of HF patients with concomitant kidney disease, making it difficult to draw conclusions regarding the effectiveness of HF medications in this population. The available evidence from RCTs provides support for the use of ACE inhibitors, ARBs, and beta-blockers in patients with mild to moderate kidney disease. Treatment with aldosterone antagonists may also be beneficial. In all cases, the serum creatinine and potassium concentrations must be carefully monitored to prevent adverse effects, as the safety of these medications in patients with moderate to severe kidney disease remains largely untested. Data for patients with HF and ESRD on dialysis are even sparser, although treatment with beta-blockers and perhaps an ACE-I or ARB is warranted. The relative paucity of data underscores the need for future RCTs of HF to include patients across all levels of kidney disease, because this special population, at high risk for poor clinical outcomes and adverse medication side effects, may also have the most to gain from effective treatment strategies.

CONCLUDING REMARKS

CER is a key component to improving HF management. Many patients in clinical practice are dissimilar to the patients in RCTs, so alternative sources of information must guide treatment. There is reasonable evidence to support the use of most HF therapeutics in women but less evidence to support use in elderly patients and patients with kidney disease. Safety issues are of particular concern in these special populations.

The American Recovery and Reinvestment Act of 2009 marked a milestone in clinical research by allocating $1.1 billion for CER.[5] The expansion of electronic medical records and statistical methods, in conjunction with this new source of funding, will create opportunities to study HF outcomes in special populations and provide more evidence to improve management strategies in these vulnerable patients with HF.

REFERENCES

1. Simon R. Patient subsets and variation in therapeutic efficacy. Br J Clin Pharmacol 1982;14(4):473–82.
2. Lloyd-Jones D, Adams RJ, Brown TM, et al. Heart disease and stroke statistics–2010 update: a report from the American Heart Association. Circulation 2010;121(7):e46–215.
3. Heiat A, Gross CP, Krumholz HM. Representation of the elderly, women, and minorities in heart failure clinical trials. Arch Intern Med 2002;162(15):1682–8.
4. Masoudi FA, Havranek EP, Wolfe P, et al. Most hospitalized older persons do not meet the enrollment criteria for clinical trials in heart failure. Am Heart J 2003;146(2):250–7.
5. Sox HC, Greenfield S. Comparative effectiveness research: a report from the Institute of Medicine. Ann Intern Med 2009;151(3):203–5.
6. Wang R, Lagakos SW, Ware JH, et al. Statistics in medicine–reporting of subgroup analyses in clinical trials. N Engl J Med 2007;357(21):2189–94.
7. Schneeweiss S, Rassen JA, Glynn RJ, et al. High-dimensional propensity score adjustment in studies of treatment effects using health care claims data. Epidemiology 2009;20(4):512–22.
8. Brookhart MA, Schneeweiss S, Rothman KJ, et al. Variable selection for propensity score models. Am J Epidemiol 2006;163(12):1149–56.
9. D'Agostino RB Jr. Propensity scores in cardiovascular research. Circulation 2007;115(17):2340–3.
10. Shah RU, Klein L, Lloyd-Jones DM. Heart failure in women: epidemiology, biology and treatment. Womens Health 2009;5(5):517–27.
11. Hsich EM, Pina IL. Heart failure in women: a need for prospective data. J Am Coll Cardiol 2009;54(6):491–8.
12. Anonymous. Effect of metoprolol CR/XL in chronic heart failure: Metoprolol CR/XL Randomised Intervention Trial in Congestive Heart Failure (MERIT-HF). Lancet 1999;353(9169):2001–7.
13. Ghali JK, Pina IL, Gottlieb SS, et al. Metoprolol CR/XL in female patients with heart failure: analysis of the experience in Metoprolol Extended-Release Randomized Intervention Trial in Heart Failure (MERIT-HF). Circulation 2002;105(13):1585–91.
14. Packer M, Bristow MR, Cohn JN, et al. The effect of carvedilol on morbidity and mortality in patients with chronic heart failure. U.S. Carvedilol Heart Failure Study Group. N Engl J Med 1996;334(21):1349–55.
15. Packer M, Coats AJ, Fowler MB, et al. Effect of carvedilol on survival in severe chronic heart failure. N Engl J Med 2001;344(22):1651–8.
16. Shekelle PG, Rich MW, Morton SC, et al. Efficacy of angiotensin-converting enzyme inhibitors and beta-blockers in the management of left ventricular systolic dysfunction according to race, gender, and diabetic status: a meta-analysis of major clinical trials. J Am Coll Cardiol 2003;41(9):1529–38.
17. Keyhan G, Chen SF, Pilote L. The effectiveness of beta-blockers in women with congestive heart failure. J Gen Intern Med 2007;22(7):955–61.
18. Hernandez AF, Hammill BG, O'Connor CM, et al. Clinical effectiveness of beta-blockers in heart failure: findings from the OPTIMIZE-HF (Organized Program to Initiate Lifesaving Treatment in Hospitalized Patients with Heart Failure) Registry. J Am Coll Cardiol 2009;53(2):184–92.
19. Keyhan G, Chen SF, Pilote L. Angiotensin-converting enzyme inhibitors and survival in women and men with heart failure. Eur J Heart Fail 2007;9(6–7):594–601.
20. Pfeffer MA, Swedberg K, Granger CB, et al. Effects of candesartan on mortality and morbidity in patients with chronic heart failure: the CHARM-Overall programme [Erratum appears in Lancet 2009

Nov 21–2009 Nov 27;(9703):1744]. Lancet 2003; 362(9386):759–66.

21. Pitt B, Zannad F, Remme WJ, et al. The effect of spironolactone on morbidity and mortality in patients with severe heart failure. Randomized Aldactone Evaluation Study Investigators. N Engl J Med 1999;341(10):709–17.

22. Pitt B, Remme W, Zannad F, et al. Eplerenone, a selective aldosterone blocker, in patients with left ventricular dysfunction after myocardial infarction. N Engl J Med 2003;348(14):1309–21.

23. Zannad F, McMurray JJV, van Veldhuisen DJ, et al. Eplerenone in patients with systolic heart failure and mild symptoms. N Engl J Med 2011;364(1): 11–21.

24. Anonymous. The effect of digoxin on mortality and morbidity in patients with heart failure. The Digitalis Investigation Group. N Engl J Med 1997;336(8): 525–33.

25. Rathore SS, Wang Y, Krumholz HM, et al. Sex-based differences in the effect of digoxin for the treatment of heart failure. N Engl J Med 2002; 347(18):1403–11.

26. Ahmed A, Rich MW, Love TE, et al. Digoxin and reduction in mortality and hospitalization in heart failure: a comprehensive post hoc analysis of the DIG trial. Eur Heart J 2006;27(2):178–86.

27. Zhou J, Shi H, Zhang J, et al. Rationale and design of the [beta]-blocker in heart failure with normal left ventricular ejection fraction (β-PRESERVE) study. Eur J Heart Fail 2010;12(2):181–5.

28. Aldosterone Antagonist Therapy for Adults With Heart Failure and Preserved Systolic Function (TOP-CAT). 2011. Available at: http://clinicaltrials.gov/ct2/show/NCT00094302. Accessed January 11, 2011.

29. Diastolic Heart Failure Management by Nifedipine (DEMAND). Available at: http://clinicaltrials.gov/ct2/show/NCT01157481. Accessed January 11, 2011.

30. Senni M, Tribouilloy CM, Rodeheffer RJ, et al. Congestive heart failure in the community: trends in incidence and survival in a 10-year period. Arch Intern Med 1999;159(1):29–34.

31. Curtis LH, Whellan DJ, Hammill BG, et al. Incidence and prevalence of heart failure in elderly persons, 1994-2003. Arch Intern Med 2008;168(4):418–24.

32. Deedwania PC, Gottlieb S, Ghali JK, et al. Efficacy, safety and tolerability of beta-adrenergic blockade with metoprolol CR/XL in elderly patients with heart failure. Eur Heart J 2004;25(15):1300–9.

33. Krum H, Hill J, Fruhwald F, et al. Tolerability of beta-blockers in elderly patients with chronic heart failure: the COLA II study. Eur J Heart Fail 2006;8(3):302–7.

34. Flather MD, Shibata MC, Coats AJS, et al. Randomized trial to determine the effect of nebivolol on mortality and cardiovascular hospital admission in elderly patients with heart failure (SENIORS). Eur Heart J 2005;26(3):215–25.

35. Flather MD, Yusuf S, Kober L, et al. Long-term ACE-inhibitor therapy in patients with heart failure or left-ventricular dysfunction: a systematic overview of data from individual patients. ACE-Inhibitor Myocardial Infarction Collaborative Group. Lancet 2000; 355(9215):1575–81.

36. Masoudi FA, Rathore SS, Wang Y, et al. National patterns of use and effectiveness of angiotensin-converting enzyme inhibitors in older patients with heart failure and left ventricular systolic dysfunction. Circulation 2004;110(6):724–31.

37. Masoudi FA, Krumholz HM. Polypharmacy and co-morbidity in heart failure. BMJ 2003;327(7414): 513–4.

38. Shlipak MG, Massie BM. The clinical challenge of cardiorenal syndrome. Circulation 2004;110(12): 1514–7.

39. Dinsdale C, Wani M, Steward J, et al. Tolerability of spironolactone as adjunctive treatment for heart failure in patients over 75 years of age. Age Ageing 2005;34(4):395–8.

40. Juurlink DN, Mamdani MM, Lee DS, et al. Rates of hyperkalemia after publication of the Randomized Aldactone Evaluation Study. N Engl J Med 2004; 351(6):543–51.

41. Heywood JT, Fonarow GC, Costanzo MR, et al. High prevalence of renal dysfunction and its impact on outcome in 118,465 patients hospitalized with acute decompensated heart failure: a report from the ADHERE database. J Card Fail 2007;13(6): 422–30.

42. McAlister FA, Ezekowitz J, Tonelli M, et al. Renal insufficiency and heart failure: prognostic and therapeutic implications from a prospective cohort study. Circulation 2004;109(8):1004–9.

43. Smith GL, Lichtman JH, Bracken MB, et al. Renal impairment and outcomes in heart failure: systematic review and meta-analysis. J Am Coll Cardiol 2006;47(10):1987–96.

44. Dries DL, Exner DV, Domanski MJ, et al. The prognostic implications of renal insufficiency in asymptomatic and symptomatic patients with left ventricular systolic dysfunction. J Am Coll Cardiol 2000;35(3):681–9.

45. Anand IS, Bishu K, Rector TS, et al. Proteinuria, chronic kidney disease, and the effect of an angiotensin receptor blocker in addition to an angiotensin-converting enzyme inhibitor in patients with moderate to severe heart failure. Circulation 2009;120(16):1577–84.

46. Shlipak MG, Smith GL, Rathore SS, et al. Renal function, digoxin therapy, and heart failure outcomes: evidence from the digoxin intervention group trial. J Am Soc Nephrol 2004;15(8): 2195–203.

47. Hjalmarson A, Goldstein S, Fagerberg B, et al. Effects of controlled-release metoprolol on total

mortality, hospitalizations, and well-being in patients with heart failure: the Metoprolol CR/XL Randomized Intervention Trial in congestive heart failure (MERIT-HF). MERIT-HF Study Group. JAMA 2000;283(10): 1295–302.

48. Ghali JK, Wikstrand J, Van Veldhuisen DJ, et al. The influence of renal function on clinical outcome and response to beta-blockade in systolic heart failure: insights from Metoprolol CR/XL Randomized Intervention Trial in Chronic HF (MERIT-HF). J Card Fail 2009;15(4):310–8.

49. Anonymous. The Cardiac Insufficiency Bisoprolol Study II (CIBIS-II): a randomised trial. Lancet 1999; 353(9146):9–13.

50. Erdmann E, Lechat P, Verkenne P, et al. Results from post-hoc analyses of the CIBIS II trial: effect of bisoprolol in high-risk patient groups with chronic heart failure. Eur J Heart Fail 2001;3(4):469–79.

51. Cohen-Solal A, Kotecha D, van Veldhuisen DJ, et al. Efficacy and safety of nebivolol in elderly heart failure patients with impaired renal function: insights from the SENIORS trial. Eur J Heart Fail 2009;11(9): 872–80.

52. Cice G, Di Benedetto A, D'Isa S, et al. Effects of telmisartan added to angiotensin-converting enzyme inhibitors on mortality and morbidity in hemodialysis patients with chronic heart failure: a double-blind, placebo-controlled trial. J Am Coll Cardiol 2010; 56(21):1701–8.

53. Anonymous. Effect of enalapril on survival in patients with reduced left ventricular ejection fractions and congestive heart failure. The SOLVD Investigators. N Engl J Med 1991;325(5):293–302.

54. Anonymous. Effects of enalapril on mortality in severe congestive heart failure. Results of the Cooperative North Scandinavian Enalapril Survival Study (CONSENSUS). The CONSENSUS Trial Study Group. N Engl J Med 1987;316(23):1429–35.

55. Konstam MA, Neaton JD, Dickstein K, et al. Effects of high-dose versus low-dose losartan on clinical outcomes in patients with heart failure (HEAAL study): a randomised, double-blind trial. Lancet 2009;374(9704):1840–8.

56. Takahashi A, Takase H, Toriyama T, et al. Candesartan, an angiotensin II type-1 receptor blocker, reduces cardiovascular events in patients on chronic haemodialysis–a randomized study. Nephrol Dial Transplant 2006;21(9):2507–12.

57. Suzuki H, Kanno Y, Sugahara S, et al. Effect of angiotensin receptor blockers on cardiovascular events in patients undergoing hemodialysis: an open-label randomized controlled trial. Am J Kidney Dis 2008;52(3):501–6.

58. Cohn JN, Tognoni G, Valsartan Heart Failure Trial I. A randomized trial of the angiotensin-receptor blocker valsartan in chronic heart failure. N Engl J Med 2001;345(23):1667–75.

59. McMurray JJV, Ostergren J, Swedberg K, et al. Effects of candesartan in patients with chronic heart failure and reduced left-ventricular systolic function taking angiotensin-converting-enzyme inhibitors: the CHARM-Added trial. Lancet 2003;362(9386):767–71.

60. Bakris G, Vassalotti J, Ritz E, et al. National Kidney Foundation consensus conference on cardiovascular and kidney diseases and diabetes risk: an integrated therapeutic approach to reduce events. Kidney Int 2010;78(8):726–36.

61. Anonymous. Effect of enalapril on mortality and the development of heart failure in asymptomatic patients with reduced left ventricular ejection fractions. The SOLVD Investigators. N Engl J Med 1992;327(10):685–91.

62. Ljungman S, Kjekshus J, Swedberg K. Renal function in severe congestive heart failure during treatment with enalapril (the Cooperative North Scandinavian Enalapril Survival Study [CONSENSUS] Trial). Am J Cardiol 1992;70(4):479–87.

63. Granger CB, McMurray JJ, Yusuf S, et al. Effects of candesartan in patients with chronic heart failure and reduced left-ventricular systolic function intolerant to angiotensin-converting-enzyme inhibitors: the CHARM-Alternative trial. Lancet 2003;362(9386):772–6.

64. Pitt B, Segal R, Martinez FA, et al. Randomised trial of losartan versus captopril in patients over 65 with heart failure (Evaluation of Losartan in the Elderly Study, ELITE). Lancet 1997;349(9054):747–52.

65. Wei L, Struthers AD, Fahey T, et al. Spironolactone use and renal toxicity: population based longitudinal analysis. BMJ 2010;340:c1768.

66. Hunt SA, Abraham WT, Chin MH, et al. 2009 focused update incorporated into the ACC/AHA 2005 Guidelines for the Diagnosis and Management of Heart Failure in Adults: a report of the American College of Cardiology Foundation/American Heart Association Task Force on Practice Guidelines. Circulation 2009;119(14):e391–479.

67. The International Steering Committee on Behalf of the MERIT-HF Study Group. Rationale, Design, and Organization of the Metoprolol CR/XL Randomized Intervention Trial in Heart Failure (MERIT-HF). Am J Cardiol 1997;80(9 Suppl 2):54J–8J.

68. Shibata MC, Flather MD, Bohm M, et al. Study of the Effects of Nebivolol Intervention on Outcomes and Rehospitalisation in Seniors with Heart Failure (SENIORS). Rationale and design. Int J Cardiol 2002;86(1):77–85.

69. Poole-Wilson PA, Swedberg K, Cleland JG, et al. Comparison of carvedilol and metoprolol on clinical outcomes in patients with chronic heart failure in the Carvedilol Or Metoprolol European Trial (COMET): randomised controlled trial. Lancet 2003;362(9377): 7–13.

70. Poole-Wilson PA, Cleland JG, Di Lenarda A, et al. Rationale and design of the carvedilol or metoprolol

European trial in patients with chronic heart failure: COMET. Eur J Heart Fail 2002;4(3):321–9.

71. Anonymous. Effect of ramipril on mortality and morbidity of survivors of acute myocardial infarction with clinical evidence of heart failure. The Acute Infarction Ramipril Efficacy (AIRE) Study Investigators. Lancet 1993;342(8875):821–8.

72. Hall AS, Winter C, Bogle SM, et al. The Acute Infarction Ramipril Efficacy (AIRE) Study: rationale, design, organization, and outcome definitions. J Cardiovasc Pharmacol 1991;18(Suppl 2): S105–9.

73. Ambrosioni E, Borghi C, Magnani B. The effect of the angiotensin-converting-enzyme inhibitor zofenopril on mortality and morbidity after anterior myocardial infarction. The Survival of Myocardial Infarction Long-Term Evaluation (SMILE) Study Investigators. N Engl J Med 1995;332(2):80–5.

74. Kober L, Torp-Pedersen C, Carlsen JE, et al. A clinical trial of the angiotensin-converting-enzyme inhibitor trandolapril in patients with left ventricular dysfunction after myocardial infarction. Trandolapril Cardiac Evaluation (TRACE) Study Group. N Engl J Med 1995;333(25):1670–6.

75. Pfeffer MA, Braunwald E, Moye LA, et al. Effect of captopril on mortality and morbidity in patients with left ventricular dysfunction after myocardial infarction. Results of the survival and ventricular enlargement trial. The SAVE Investigators. N Engl J Med 1992;327(10):669–77.

The Economics of Heart Failure

Dhruv S. Kazi, MD, MSc, MS[a], Daniel B. Mark, MD, MPH[b],*

KEYWORDS

- Heart failure • Economics • Therapies • Cost-effectiveness • Quality-adjusted life years

KEY POINTS

- The overall annual US medical spending attributed to heart failure is approximately $39 billion.
- Making choices based on the relative efficiency with which therapies improve health is rational, although issues besides rationality often need to be included in decision making.
- Angiotensin-converting enzyme inhibitors, β-blockers, aldosterone antagonists, and implantable cardioverter-defibrillators are cost-effective by conventional criteria in patients with systolic heart failure.
- In appropriately selected patients with advanced heart failure, the use of cardiac resynchronization therapy (CRT) devices without defibrillation capabilities (CRT-P) as well as heart transplantation seems to provide good value for money.
- The relative effectiveness and cost-effectiveness of CRT devices with defibrillation capabilities (relative to CRT-P devices) and left ventricular assist devices remain uncertain.

BACKGROUND

At 17% of the gross domestic product, the US health care system is the most expensive in the world, and its per capita expenditure on health care is more than twice the average of other developed countries (**Fig. 1**).[1] Although generally considered to be a private (vs a public) system, health care spending in the United States is a large and growing share of government budgets, presently accounting for about one-quarter of total federal spending. The nonpartisan Congressional Budget Office projects that, under current policies, health care spending will account for almost one-half of all federal noninterest outlays by 2050.[2]

Statistics to show that heart failure is an expensive disease are easy to come by. There are an estimated 1 million heart failure hospitalizations each year, and heart failure is the most common indication for hospitalization among Medicare enrollees. The overall annual US medical spending attributed to heart failure is approximately $39 billion.[3] What is less clear is the extent to which those costs can be reduced while maintaining high-quality care and supporting innovation. The Patient Protection and Affordable Care Act passed by the US Congress in March 2010 emphasizes the need to rein in US health care costs but explicitly excludes cost considerations from policy making.[4] In making this specification, Congress was attempting to avoid any accusations of rationing care by cost. What Congress perhaps failed to understand is that making choices is unavoidable in a world in which it is unaffordable to provide all possibly useful care to everyone. Making choices based on the relative efficiency with which therapies improve health is rational, although issues besides rationality often need to be included in decision making. Medical economics is a discipline that provides conceptual

Funding Source: Funded in part by an American Heart Association-Pharmaceutical Round Table Cardiovascular Outcomes Research fellowship to D.S.K.

a Division of Cardiology, Department of Medicine, University of California, 1001 Potrero Ave, 5G1, San Francisco, CA 94110, USA; b Outcomes Research Group, Duke Clinical Research Institute, Duke University Medical Center, 2400 Pratt Avenue, Room 0311, Durham, NC 27707, USA
* Corresponding author. PO Box 17969, Durham, NC 27715.
E-mail address: daniel.mark@duke.edu

Heart Failure Clin 9 (2013) 93–106
http://dx.doi.org/10.1016/j.hfc.2012.09.005
1551-7136/13/$ – see front matter © 2013 Elsevier Inc. All rights reserved.

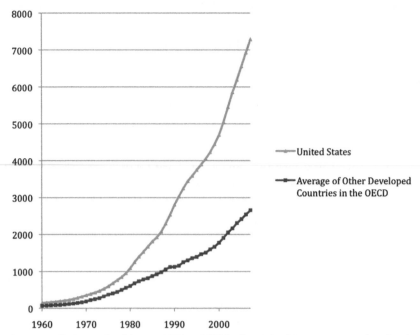

Fig. 1. Per capita expenditures on health care 1960 to 2007 in the United States versus other developed countries in the Organization for Economic Co-operation and Development (OECD). (*Data from* Health Data 2010: Statistics and Indicators. 2010. Available at: http://www.oecd.org/document/30/0,3746,en_2649_37407_12968734_1_1_1_37407,00.html. Accessed December 21, 2010.)

and quantitative tools to address the problem of allocating scarce resources efficiently. This article discusses some of the general concepts of health economics and provides a brief review of economic outcomes of heart failure therapies.

HEALTH ECONOMICS 101

The central axiom of economics is that resources are scarce and wants are unlimited. Any resources committed to health care are no longer available for other uses. In the classic guns-versus-butter trade-off from freshman economics, the decision to produce more weapons (defense spending) means that fewer resources are available for food production or other societal priorities such as health care. Economics does not offer any advice on whether it is better to produce more weapons or more food or more medical care; this is ultimately a policy decision and therefore outside the formal purview of economics. However, economics can provide information on the relative efficiency of each possible investment being considered.

From the perspective of the economist, cost is therefore not an amount of money but rather the consumption of societal resources that are then lost to any other use. What is considered a cost varies substantially based on whose perspective is being considered. For example, from a societal

perspective, a readmission for heart failure intuitively is an added cost to the system. From the perspective of an insured patient, the incremental cost may equal a copay, which is a tiny fraction of the total cost of the hospitalization. From the perspective of the hospital administrator or the treating physician, a readmission may represent additional revenue (under current reimbursement policies in a fee-for-service system). When examining the health economic literature, the perspective used by the investigators is relevant to the interpretation of reported results.

Another important issue in economic analyses is the time horizon being considered. The time horizon ideally should fully encompass all the consequences of the initial resource allocation decision being studied. Thus, if it is decided to implant a primary prevention implantable cardioverter-defibrillator (ICD) in a patient with heart failure, the cost analysis of such a strategy needs to consider not only the initial costs of the ICD implantation but also the long-term costs of care for complications, generator replacements, and upgrades for the lifetime of the patient.

COST-EFFECTIVENESS ANALYSES

Cost-effectiveness analysis is a method of comparing incremental benefits and costs. Incremental in this context means added to what already exists. For example, the decision to treat a patient who has coronary artery disease with coronary artery bypass grafting (CABG) means that the costs of the surgery are incremental to the costs of the medical therapy that the patient would receive with or without the surgery. Surgery does not replace evidence-based medical therapy; it is added to such therapy. The important concept here is that economic analyses need to measure costs that are incremental, whereas costs that are the same in the 2 treatment options being considered cancel out and are not considered further.

In general, 2 types of cost-effectiveness analyses are commonly encountered in the medical literature: those based on randomized clinical trials (RCT) and those based on decision-analytical modeling (DAM). In the former, cost and outcomes data are prospectively collected alongside clinical data while conducting an RCT. As with clinical data, the costs and quality-adjusted life years (QALYs) estimated from an RCT may provide an objective measure of the impact of the intervention being studied. However, this method of cost-effectiveness analysis has several important limitations. The costs incurred in an RCT are likely influenced by the characteristics of the patients recruited to the study (who are generally younger and healthier than patients in the reference patient population) as well as the clinical centers where the trial is being conducted (often academic centers that have greater clinical expertise but higher costs). More importantly, RCTs tend to have short durations of follow-up (eg, the longest trial data available for cardiac resynchronization is less than 3 years of follow-up) and therefore cannot directly provide estimates of lifetime costs or benefits.

These limitations can be overcome by the use of decision-analytical modeling, wherein investigators design a mathematical model to recreate the natural history of a disease. The model incorporates average outcomes from published RCTs, or meta-analyses thereof, and average costs from published tariffs or resource-use studies. A distinct advantage of this method is the ability to test the robustness of the results by subjecting the model to rigorous sensitivity analyses in which 1 or more input parameters are varied, individually or simultaneously, to test how this influences the reported results.

An example can serve to show some of the key concepts involved in cost-effectiveness analyses. The value of a new technology such as cardiac resynchronization therapy (CRT) can be judged by comparing it with a relevant therapeutic alternative (eg, optimal pharmacologic therapy and calculating the incremental cost-effectiveness ratio (ICER). The ICER is the total net cost of the new therapy compared with the alternative therapy, divided by the total net effectiveness of the new therapy compared with the alternative:

$$ICER = \frac{Cost_{NewTherapy} - Cost_{Alternative}}{Outcomes_{NewTherapy} - Outcomes_{Alternative}}$$

In estimating *ICERs*, costs are generally measured in monetary terms (eg, dollar value of the resources used). Quantifying clinical outcomes in monetary terms, as in cost-benefit analysis, is more problematic (how many dollars is 1 life year worth?), so these are often reported using the simple but imperfect unit of life years or QALYs.[5]

Several key concepts of health economics emerge from this simple equation.

First, cost-effectiveness is measured in incremental terms and therefore requires the identification of an appropriate comparator. If no standard of care exists, the comparator may be placebo or usual care. If multiple alternatives exist, each strategy must be compared with the next best alternative. The choice of comparator is a significant determinant of the estimated ICER.

The second concept is perhaps the most important: a therapy must be effective before it can be cost-effective. Economic evaluations must therefore begin with comprehensive evaluations of clinical effectiveness (and stop there, if no such evidence exists). Hence the assertion that health economics research is a comprehensive form of comparative effectiveness research and that there can be no inherent tension between the two.[6]

Third, because both costs and outcomes of a disease change with time, a cost-effectiveness study must capture all relevant costs and outcomes over the relevant time horizon (**Fig. 2**). For instance, CRT for advanced symptomatic heart failure results in substantial up-front costs of implanting the device (~$40,000) and possible perioperative morbidity and mortality, but its benefits accrue over the ensuing years. The up-front costs of the device and its implantation may be offset over time by the costs saved by preventing heart failure hospitalizations. Thus, analyzing costs and outcomes at the 12-month mark would provide an unrealistic (and falsely unfavorable) ICER. A 6-year analysis may also provide a biased estimate, given the average battery life of 7 to 8 years and the costs and morbidity associated with a generator change. Wherever possible, costs and outcomes must be analyzed over the lifetime of the patients, and any deviations from this must be carefully scrutinized.

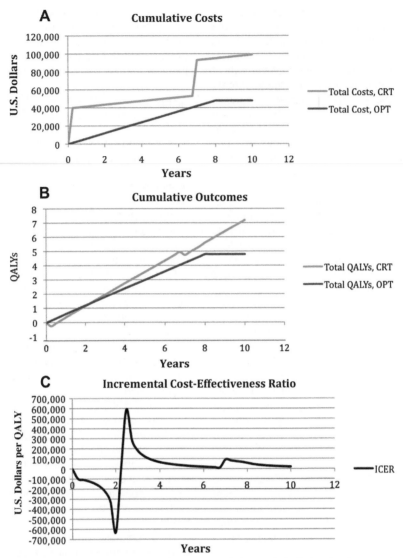

Fig. 2. A hypothetical scenario to demonstrate the impact of the analytical time horizon on incremental cost-effectiveness. *(A)* Cumulative costs, US Dollars. *(B)* Cumulative outcomes (quality-adjusted life years, QALYs). *(C)* Incremental cost-effectiveness ratio (ICER) at various time points (US Dollars per QALY). Consider 2 identical cohorts of patients with advanced symptomatic heart failure. One cohort receives cardiac resynchronization therapy (CRT) at time 0, whereas the other is managed on optimal pharmacologic therapy alone (OPT). The cohort receiving CRT faces the costs *(A)* and QALY penalties *(B)* associated with initial device implantation at year 0 and generator change at year 7. However, as a result of cardiac resynchronization, the CRT cohort has improved quality-of-life (due to improvement in symptoms), increased life expectancy (due to fewer heart failure deaths), and lower costs (due to fewer heart failure hospitalizations). Panel C shows the dynamic nature of the ICER. In this hypothetical example, CRT costs more and generates fewer QALYs in the first two years (dominated, or clearly inferior). Beyond year 4, CRT generates more QALYs than OPT, which justifies the high upfront costs. CRT therefore appears to be cost-effective at a threshold of $100,000/QALY. Note the significant increase in the ICER at year 7, when the need for a generator change incurs substantial costs and QALY penalties. Thus the ICER for cardiac resynchronization relative to medical therapy alone is highly dependent on how long patients are followed for. Arbitrarily truncating the analysis at any point before death produces a biased estimate of the ICER. A lifetime analytical horizon is therefore most appropriate. Undiscounted costs and QALYs depicted for simplicity; see text for details.

This article reviews selected studies of various diagnostic and therapeutic interventions in patients with heart failure, including RCT-based and DAM-based analyses.

COST-EFFECTIVENESS IN HEART FAILURE
Diagnostic Strategies in Heart Failure

Natriuretic peptide levels are now routinely used in the management of patients presenting to the emergency room with acute dyspnea.[7,8] Mueller and colleagues[9] prospectively collected data on resource use alongside an RCT to estimate the cost-effectiveness of B-type natriuretic peptide (BNP)–guided management of patients presenting to the emergency room with dyspnea. BNP testing resulted in several important changes in the management of these patients, including reductions in initial hospital admission rate, use of intensive care, and total inpatient days at 180 days. Patients in the BNP-guided group had a significantly lower total treatment cost relative to patients in the usual care arm ($7930 vs $10,503; $P = .004$). To estimate the degree of uncertainty in the incremental cost-effectiveness, the investigators performed 5000 bootstrap replications (resampling with replacement to assess the variance of the ICER); BNP guidance resulted in lower mortality and lower cost in 80.6% of these replications.

Heidenreich and colleagues[10] developed a Markov model to examine the role of BNP in screening asymptomatic members of the general population for left ventricular systolic dysfunction. In their model, patients with an increased BNP underwent a subsequent transthoracic echo to evaluate cardiac function. In this model, screening 1000 asymptomatic patients increased the lifetime cost of care ($176,000 for men; $101,000 for women) but improved outcomes (7.9 additional QALYs for men, 1.3 QALYs for women), resulting in a cost per QALY of $22,300 for men and $77,700 for women. The ICER was less than $50,000 per QALY for populations in which the prevalence of left ventricular systolic dysfunction was 1% or greater.[10] However, this strategy has not gained much acceptance in the cardiology or public health communities, partly because subsequent studies have shown that BNP screening is a suboptimal tool for detecting asymptomatic left ventricular systolic dysfunction.[11]

Medical Therapy

β-Blockers
The recognition of the maladaptive role of the adrenergic system in chronic heart failure and the role of β-blockade in the management of

chronic systolic heart failure represented considerable progress in understanding the pathophysiology of the disease and its management.[12] A series of landmark trials showed that β-blocker therapy reduces the risk of hospitalization for heart failure and all-cause mortality in patients with mild to severe systolic heart failure.[13–17] Although it is possible that the benefits of β-blockers may be a class effect, it should be noted that the drugs that have been shown to unequivocally improve outcomes in chronic systolic heart failure are bisoprolol, carvedilol, and metoprolol succinate.

The efficacy of carvedilol was shown in the US Carvedilol Heart Failure Trials Program, involving 4 concurrent, randomized, double-blind, placebo-controlled trials in 1094 patients with New York Heart Association (NYHA) class II to IV symptoms and left ventricular ejection fraction (LVEF) less than or equal to 0.35.[15] The program was terminated early based on a finding of a 65% reduction in the risk of mortality in patients receiving carvedilol (95% confidence interval [CI], 39%–80%), and a 53% reduction in the mean number of chronic heart failure-related hospitalizations (CI, 19%–70%).[18] Delea and colleagues[18] used these data to design a Markov decision model to evaluate the impact of carvedilol over the lifetime of patients with systolic heart failure. Assuming that the benefits of carvedilol last 6 months (the average duration of the trials) and then gradually decline to zero over the next 2.5 years, carvedilol was estimated to improve life expectancy by 0.95 years (from 6.67 to 7.62 years) at an incremental lifetime cost (in 1997 US dollars) of $15,735. Given that generic versions of carvedilol can now be obtained for as little as $10 for a 3-month supply at leading pharmacies in the United States, it would be expected that carvedilol now has an ICER that is more favorable than the $19,918 per discounted life year saved reported from this model. Moreover, the increasing costs of medical care (such as heart failure hospitalizations) should further depress the estimated ICER. Thus, carvedilol seems to be cost-effective in patients with systolic heart failure.

Bisoprolol and metoprolol succinate have also been shown to improve survival in chronic heart failure; however, no US economic analyses are available. Cost-effectiveness analyses from the perspective of other countries have suggested favorable results.[19,20]

Angiotensin-converting enzyme inhibitors
Drugs that inhibit the angiotensin-converting enzyme (ACE) are a cornerstone of drug therapy for systolic heart failure, improving survival, and reducing hospitalizations.[21] Several RCT-based

and DAM-based economic analyses have shown that the use of ACE inhibitors in heart failure is extremely cost-effective. For example, Glick and colleagues[22,23] examined the cost-effectiveness of enalapril using data from the Studies of Left Ventricular Dysfunction (SOLVD) treatment trial, which randomized 2569 patients with symptomatic systolic heart failure (with LVEF $\leq$0.35) to receive either enalapril or placebo. Estimating costs and QALYs over the patients' lifetimes, the investigators found that the use of enalapril produced a survival benefit of 0.40 years at an incremental cost of $80 per year of life saved and $115 per QALY saved. As noted in the case of carvedilol, generic versions of ACE inhibitors are now widely available on the market, making it likely that enalapril is now cost saving in patients with symptomatic systolic heart failure.[6]

Angiotensin receptor blockers

By directly binding with the angiotensin receptors, angiotensin receptor blockers (ARBs) act as potent inhibitors of the renin-angiotensin system and circumvent the problem of chronic cough associated with ACE inhibitors attributed to the increased accumulation of bradykinin (which is also degraded by ACE). The role of ARB therapy in chronic systolic heart failure has been evaluated both as an adjunct to and a substitute for ACE inhibitors. Relative to placebo, ARBs have been associated with reduced all-cause mortality (odds ratio [OR] 0.83; CI 0.69–1.00) and heart failure hospitalizations (OR, 0.64 [CI, 0.53 to 0.78]); in contrast, relative to ACE inhibitors, all-cause mortality (OR 1.06; CI 0.90–1.26) and heart failure hospitalization (OR 0.95; CI 0.80–1.13) did not differ.[24] In addition, in the comparison of the combination of ARBs plus ACE inhibitors versus ACE inhibitors alone, all-cause mortality was not reduced (OR 0.97; CI 0.87–1.08) despite a significant reduction in heart failure hospitalizations (OR 0.77; CI 0.69–0.87).

While commenting on the efficacy of ARBs, it is important to emphasize that one of the first large RCTs to specifically address patients with heart failure and preserved LVEF was an ARB versus placebo trial. In CHARM-Preserved (the preserved LVEF arm of the Candesartan in Heart Failure: Assessment of Reduction in Mortality and Morbidity program), Yusuf and colleagues[25] randomized 3023 patients with chronic heart failure and LVEF greater than 0.4 to candesartan or placebo. With a median follow-up of 36.6 months, there was a trend to improvement in the composite end point of cardiovascular death or admission to hospital for chronic heart failure (co-variate-adjusted hazard ratio 0·86; CI 0·74–1·0;

P = 0.051). Although cardiovascular death did not differ between groups, fewer patients experienced 1 or more hospitalizations for heart failure in the candesartan arm.

There are no available economic analyses from a US perspective comparing ARBs with placebo or with ACE inhibitors in patients with heart failure. An economic analysis from a European perspective of the CHARM program reported that the cost of the medication is largely offset by the savings associated with decreased heart failure hospitalizations. In ACE-intolerant patients with an ejection fraction less than or equal to 0.40, the use of candesartan is cost saving and achieves dominance compared with placebo.[26]

Isosorbide-hydralazine

The isosorbide-hydralazine combination studied in the African American Heart Failure Trial (A-HeFT) showed a decrease in the risk of all-cause mortality (10.2% vs 6.2%) in black patients with symptomatic heart failure and depressed systolic function (LVEF $\leq$0.35, or LVEF <0.45 and left ventricular end diastolic dimension >6.5 cm).[27] Angus and colleagues[28] prospectively collected resource-use data with this trial to estimate the cost-effectiveness of the fixed-dose isosorbide-hydralazine combination. At a drug cost of $6 a day, the use of isosorbide-hydralazine combination reduced heart failure–related expenditures and improved outcomes over the course of the trial (mean follow-up, 12.8 months). From a lifetime analytical horizon, the combination had an ICER of $44,400/life year gained relative to placebo if its benefit was assumed to only last the duration of the trial, or $32,900/life year gained if the benefit was assumed to extend 1 year beyond the study termination. The specific proprietary combination drug studied in A-HeFT (BiDil) is no longer marketed, but generic formulations of its constituents are readily available and inexpensive, so it can be assumed that this treatment is highly cost-effective in the population studied in A-HeFT.

Digoxin

In the Digitalis Investigation Group (DIG) trial, the use of digoxin in patients with systolic heart failure conferred no survival advantage compared with placebo, but was associated with a 6% reduction in hospitalizations.[29] A now dated economic analysis based on the PROVED[30] and RADIANCE[31] studies suggested that continuing digoxin in patients with systolic heart failure would result in cost savings, provided that the rates of digoxin toxicity were less than or equal to 33%.[32] A more recent economic analysis found that the net cost of digoxin therapy over 3 years was about $160, and that the use of digoxin was cost saving in several high-risk subgroups.[33]

Aldosterone antagonists

Two aldosterone antagonists, spironolactone and eplerenone, have been shown to be effective in selected populations with heart failure. In the Randomized Aldosterone Study Investigators (RALES) trial, 1663 patients with symptomatic heart failure and LVEF less than or equal to 0.35 were randomized to spironolactone or placebo.[34] The trial was terminated early because spironolactone was associated with a 30% reduction in the risk of death (35% vs 46%; relative risk of death 0.70; CI 0.60–0.82). A decision model–based analysis of the first 35 months of the RALES trial incorporated costs from 5 countries and found that spironolactone added 0.13 QALYs and lowered costs by $713, and thus was superior to placebo.[35]

In the Eplerenone Post-Acute Myocardial Infarction Heart Failure Efficacy and Survival Study (EPHESUS), mineralocorticoid antagonism with eplerenone resulted in a 15% reduction in all-cause mortality in patients with left ventricular systolic dysfunction and heart failure after acute myocardial infarction (relative risk 0.85; CI 0.75–0.96).[36] In a cost-effectiveness analysis of EPHESUS using a lifetime analytical horizon, eplerenone added about 0.10 to 0.13 life years at an incremental cost of about $1400.[37] Using several different methods to extrapolate long-term outcomes, estimates of the ICER were consistently less than $20,000 per life year saved. In a substudy in patients previously on both an ACE inhibitor and a β-blocker, the addition of eplerenone produced an ICER less than $26,000 per QALY gained,[38] further suggesting that the use of eplerenone is economically attractive in selected patients with systolic heart failure.

The results of the EMPHASIS-HF clinical trial expanded the clinical indication for aldosterone antagonists in heart failure, previously largely limited to patients with NYHA class III heart failure.[39] In this trial, 2737 patients with NYHA class II heart failure and an LVEF less than or equal to 0.35 were randomized to receive eplerenone or placebo, in addition to standard therapy. At 21 months, eplerenone was associated with a 37% relative risk reduction in a composite of death from cardiovascular causes or hospitalization for heart failure (18.3% vs 25.9%; hazard ratio 0.63; CI 0.54–0.74). This development is significant: the use of a proprietary aldosterone antagonist in patients with NYHA class II heart failure could result in a substantial increase in prescription drug costs. However, these costs may be largely offset by the reduction in heart failure hospitalizations if the efficacy seen in the trial is reproduced in the general population.

A significant concern with the use of aldosterone antagonists is the development of hyperkalemia, including life-threatening hyperkalemia, the rates of which may be higher in the general population than those observed in clinical trials.[40] Thus an economic analysis of aldosterone antagonists based on outcomes in the general heart failure population would be informative; no such analysis is currently available.

Electrophysiologic Devices

Implantable cardioverter-defibrillators

Several clinical trials have shown the efficacy of ICDs for the primary prevention of sudden cardiac death in patients with systolic heart failure. Given the cost of the technology and the large number of patients potentially eligible for prophylactic implantation, the cost-effectiveness of these devices has been carefully examined in both RCT-based and DAM-based analyses. As would be expected, the cost-effectiveness of ICDs is sensitive to the assumption regarding the duration of protection afforded. An analysis that assumes that ICDs work only as long as the relevant clinical trial(s), and that the benefit ceases thereafter, would produce a conservative, and likely biased, estimate.[41] As shown in **Fig. 2**, the analytical time horizon significantly influences the estimated ICER of device-based therapies, and the most reliable estimates are obtained from analyses that capture lifetime costs and benefits.

A prospective economic analysis of the SCD-HeFT trial using a lifetime time horizon estimated a base case lifetime ICER of $38,389 per life year saved and $41,530 per QALY saved in moderately symptomatic patients with heart failure with LVEF less than or equal to 0.35.[42] In this study, an incremental cost-effectiveness ratio less than $100,000 per life year saved was obtained in 99% of 1000 bootstrap repetitions. However, when analyzed by NYHA class, the ICER was $29,872 per life year saved for patients with NYHA class II heart failure, whereas those with NYHA class III heart failure experienced incremental costs but no incremental benefit.

Sanders and colleagues[43] created a decision model to estimate the cost-effectiveness of ICD therapy using data from several clinical trials. In 6 of the 8 trials they examined, implantation of the ICD improved life expectancy relative to control therapy, ranging from 1.40 to 4.14 discounted years, or from 1.01 to 2.99 QALYs. The corresponding ICERs ranged from $24,500 to

$50,700 per life year added and from $34,000 to $70,200 per QALY added. However, in 2 of the trials examined (DINAMIT and Coronary Artery Bypass Graft [CABG] Patch),[44,45] patients who received an ICD had higher costs and lower life expectancy than the controls, thus the ICD was a dominated therapy in these patients. Almost entirely as a result of these trials, the prophylactic implantation of an ICD is contraindicated within 40 days after a myocardial infarction (as in DINAMIT) or at the time of surgical revascularization (as in CABG Patch). Sanders and colleagues[43] also noted that the ICER was sensitive to the assumption regarding the duration of benefit associated with the ICD; the incremental cost-effectiveness ratio was less than $100,000 per QALY as long as the ICD reduced mortality for 7 or more years.[43]

Cardiac Resynchronization Therapy

CRT represents a novel therapeutic approach to the management of advanced symptomatic heart failure and has been shown in RCT to reduce symptoms, heart failure hospitalizations, and heart failure deaths.[46–54] The economic impact of this effective but expensive therapy on total costs of care is an important consideration because the prevalence of heart failure, and the use of CRT, increases in the general population.

Two types of CRT devices are available: those with and those without defibrillation capabilities (CRT-D and CRT-P respectively). There are extensive clinical data on the efficacy of CRT-P devices relative to medical therapy alone, but there are significant additional benefits of adding the defibrillator (which nearly triples the cost) remains unclear.[55] In line with the previously discussed principles of health economics, we must first consider the cost-effectiveness of CRT-P devices relative to medical therapy, and then evaluate the incremental cost-effectiveness of CRT-D relative to CRT-P devices.

In the Cardiac Resynchronization in Heart Failure (CARE-HF) trial, 813 patients with NYHA class III or IV heart failure caused by left ventricular systolic dysfunction (LVEF <0.35) and cardiac dyssynchrony were randomized to CRT plus medical therapy versus medical therapy alone.[46] In the accompanying prospective cost-effectiveness analysis, the cost of medical care was estimated from the use of major medical resources, with unit prices based on the UK National Health Service reference costs.[56] Quality of life data were collected prospectively using validated instruments (the EQ-5D and Minnesota Living with Heart Failure Questionnaire). During a mean follow-up of 29.4 months, patients assigned to CRT had significantly increased costs (€4316; CI

1327–7485), as well as longer survival (0.10 years; CI -0.01–0.21) and improved quality of life (QALYs gained 0.22; CI, 0.13–0.32). The ICER was calculated as €19,319 per QALY gained (CI, 5482 to 45,402) and €43,596 per life year gained (CI, −146,236 to 223,849), indicating that the improvement in quality of life is an important determinant of the overall effectiveness, and hence cost-effectiveness, of this therapy. These results were sensitive to the cost of the device, implantation procedure, and heart failure hospitalization rates.

Several decision-analytical models have attempted to estimate the cost-effectiveness of CRT (**Table 1**).[57–60] Models incorporating improvements in survival as well as those in quality of life are considered here.

A Markov model based on the results of the Comparison of Medical Therapy, Pacing, and Defibrillation in Heart Failure (COMPANION) trial and with an analytical horizon of 7 years produced an incremental cost-effectiveness of $19,600 per QALY gained for CRT-P relative to medical therapy, and $160,000 per QALY gained for CRT-D relative to CRT-P,[48,58,61] suggesting that, although CRT-P is cost-effective, the addition of the defibrillator component increases the initial and long-term costs substantially, with only a modest improvement in outcomes.

Yao and colleagues[59] developed a Markov model that combined the data from the COMPANION and CARE-HF trials (CARE-HF did not have a CRT-D arm). In their model, from a lifetime perspective in a 65-year-old patient, the incremental cost-effectiveness of CRT-P relative to medical therapy was €7538 per QALY gained (CI €5325–€11,784), whereas the incremental cost-effectiveness of CRT-D relative to CRT-P was €47,909 per QALY gained (CI, €35,703–€79,438).

In a Markov model developed from the US Medicare perspective, CRT-P compared favorably with medical therapy alone using the lifetime analytical horizon, with an incremental life expectancy gain of 0.74 years and an estimated ICER of $43,378/QALY (see **Table 1**).[62] In this analysis, relative to CRT-P, CRT-D cost $34,244 more and produced 0.56 additional QALYs, resulting in an ICER of $61,114/QALY. This further underscores the need to carefully examine the value of adding the defibrillator to CRT in patients with advanced symptomatic heart failure.

Advanced Therapies for End-stage Heart Failure

Heart transplantation

For select patients with advanced refractory heart failure, heart transplantation can significantly

Table 1
Cost-effectiveness of CRT

Model	Reference	Strategy	Cost (Range, If Available)	Effect (Life Years)	Effect (QALYs)	ICER (Per Life-Year Gained)	ICER (Per QALY)	Comment
Randomized Clinical Trial:								
Analysis based on CARE-HF	56	OPT	€15,795 (3684–18,185)	1.92 (1.51–2.52)	1.19 (0.65–1.73)	—	—	Time horizon for analysis was 29.4 mo, the mean duration of follow-up in CARE-HF
		CRT-P	€20,110 (9443–22,540)	2.02 (1.62–2.53)	1.42 (1.01–1.92)	€43,596 (-146, 236–223,849)	€19,319 (5482–45,402)	
Decision Analytical Models:								
Based on Early RCTs	57	OPT	$34,400 (31,100–37,700)	—	2.64 (2.47–2.82)	—	—	Considered lifetime costs and benefits, but did not consider improvements in quality of life with CRT
		CRT-P	$64,400 (59,000–$70,200)	—	2.92 (2.72–3.14)	—	$107,800 (79,800–156,500)	
Based on COMPANION	48,58,61	OPT	$46,000	3.37	2.3	—	—	Time horizon for analysis was 7 y
		CRT-P	$59,900	3.87	3.01	$27,800[a]	$19,600[a]	
		CRT-D	$82,200	4.15	3.15	$79,600[a]	$159,200[a]	
Based on data from CARE-HF and COMPANION	59	OPT	€39,060	6.1	4.08	—	—	Considered lifetime costs and benefits
		CRT-P	€53,996	8.23	6.06	€7011 (5346–10,003)	€7538 (5325–11,784)	
		CRT-D	€87,350	9.16	6.75	€35,874 (27,709–56,353)	€47,909 (35,703–79,438)	
Based on a meta-analysis of all available RCTs	60	OPT	£9367	4.9	3.1	—	—	Considered lifetime costs and benefits
		CRT-P	£20,997	5.8	3.8	£12,922[a]	£16,735[a]	
		CRT-D	£32,687	6.2	4.09	£29,225[a]	£40,310[a]	
Uses a US Medicare perspective; based on a meta-analysis of all available RCTs	62	OPT	$14,589	4.72	3.53	—	—	Considered lifetime costs and benefits
		CRT-P	$46,255	5.46	4.26	$42,792	$43,378	
		CRT-D	$80,479	6.18	4.82	$47,533	$61,114	

This table summarizes the major cost-effectiveness analyses of cardiac resynchronization in the peer-reviewed literature, including RCT and decision analytical models. Note the variability in estimates of cost-effectiveness among the studies. The incremental cost-effectiveness ratios for CRT-P are compared with OPT, whereas the ICERs for CRT-D are compared with CRT-P. As of April 2008, $1 = €0.64 = £0.5.

Abbreviations: CRT-D, CRT with defibrillation capability; CRT-P, CRT without defibrillation capability; OPT, optimal pharmacologic therapy for heart failure; €, euros; $, Dollars (United States); £, Pounds Sterling (United Kingdom).

[a] Calculated from published data.

Adapted from Kazi D, Hlatky M. The cost-effectiveness of cardiac resynchronization therapy. In: Abraham WT, Baliga RV, editors. Cardiac resynchronization therapy in heart failure. Lippincott, Williams & Wilkins; 2009.

improve survival and enhance quality of life. With a 1-year survival rate approaching 90%, a 5-year survival rate of about 70%, and a median survival greater than 10 years, heart transplantation is a valuable therapeutic option for selected patients with end-stage heart failure.[63] Despite the benefit, the number of heart transplants conducted in the United States is small and is limited largely by the availability of donor hearts.

Heart transplantation is associated with substantial initial hospitalization costs, with single-center estimates ranging from $75,992 (in 2001)[64] to greater than $150,000 (in 2005).[65] This includes the substantial cost of procurement and transportation of the organ, in itself estimated to be about 40% of the total cost of the initial hospitalization.[64] Moreover, long-term costs of post-transplant care can be as much as $70,000 a year by some estimates, and include carefully monitored immunosuppressive therapy, periodic screening for rejection and transplant vasculopathy, and hospital admissions to treat episodes of cellular or humoral rejection.[6]

As noted previously, the cost-effectiveness of transplantation must be viewed in light of the available alternatives. Patients who do not qualify for transplants or who are unable to obtain a donor heart often have high mortality and poor quality of life. Thus the primary determinant of the cost-effectiveness of transplantation is the expected improvement in intermediate and long-term clinical outcomes. Over the past decade, refinement of donor and recipient selection methods, better donor heart management, and advances in immunosuppression have significantly improved survival.[63] Therefore, despite the high procedural and follow-up costs, it is likely that the substantial increase in life expectancy and improvement in quality of life for transplant patients makes it an economically attractive option compared with medical therapy alone in this population.

Left ventricular assist devices

Mechanical circulatory support is an evolving technology in patients with end-stage heart failure. Unlike donor hearts, the supply of left ventricular assist devices (LVADs) is potentially unlimited. However, assessing the current impact of LVAD therapy is difficult because of the rapid evolution of the technology and the expanding clinical indications for implantation. With increasing clinical experience, these artificial hearts, which were initially developed as bridge-to-transplantation therapy, are now being also used as a destination therapy for patients who do not qualify for transplantation.

As with heart transplantation, the up-front costs of this therapy are high; in 1 study, the cost of the initial hospitalization was estimated to be $198,000 (2005 estimate).[65] There is some evidence to suggest that LVAD-related costs may be decreasing with accumulating clinical experience, improvement in devices, and an increasing trend to outpatient management of patients receiving LVADs as a bridge to transplantation.[66] However, average initial costs continue to be twice as high for patients who do not survive the initial hospitalization relative to those who do, indicating the significant economic burden of device-related and non–device-related complications in these critically ill patients.[66]

Hernandez and colleagues[67] recently reported their analysis of inpatient claims for LVAD implantation among Medicare enrollees during the period 2000 to 2006. Among patients receiving the device as primary therapy (ie, excluding the patients who receive the device as a rescue strategy for postcardiotomy cardiogenic shock), only 55% were alive at discharge, and 56% of these patients were readmitted within 6 months. The overall 1-year survival was 51.6% in the primary device group, but was significantly lower after cardiotomy (30.8%). To put this in perspective, the 1-year survival for orthotopic heart transplantation is now nearly 90%. Mean 1-year Medicare payments for inpatient care for patients in the 2000 to 2005 cohorts were $178,714 ($\pm$$142,549) in the primary device group, which averaged to about $1028 per day for the first 12 months. Although informative, this analysis was limited to Medicare enrollees; costs and outcomes in younger patients, as well as privately insured patients, may differ significantly.

Given the available data, LVADs remain an expensive technology with suboptimal clinical outcomes in patients with end-stage heart failure. Despite some improvement in recent years, device-related and non-device–related complications such as mechanical failure, stroke, and infections remain significant concerns.[68,69] It is possible that, as the technology evolves and patient outcomes improve, LVADs will eventually become a clinically and economically attractive therapeutic option.[70]

Heart Failure Disease Management Programs

Multidisciplinary heart failure disease management programs have been shown to dramatically reduce heart failure hospitalizations (a major driver of costs in heart failure), and some studies have also noted an impressive survival benefit in high-risk patient populations. The impact of such programs in low-risk patients with heart failure is unclear. Chan and colleagues[71] used a Markov model to estimate the clinical and economic implications of such programs in high-risk and low-risk patients. Sensitivity analyses of various long-term scenarios took into consideration significantly reduced effectiveness in low-risk patients. The investigators reported an ICER of $9700 per life year gained and estimated that covering all patients with heart failure quadrupled life years saved compared with limiting coverage to only the highest quintile of risk. In a probabilistic sensitivity analysis, 99.74% of possible ICERs were less than $50,000 per life year gained, suggesting that heart failure disease management programs are likely cost-effective in the long term along the spectrum of patient risk.

DISCUSSION

ACE inhibitors, β-blockers, aldosterone antagonists, and ICDs are cost-effective by conventional criteria in patients with systolic heart failure. In addition, in appropriately selected patients with advanced heart failure, the use of CRT-P devices as well as heart transplantation seems to provide good value for money. In contrast, the relative effectiveness and cost-effectiveness of CRT-D devices (relative to CRT-P devices) and LVADs remain uncertain.

A few caveats regarding the application of economic principles to health care merit emphasis at this point.

The focus of health care economic evaluation is typically on health care systems and not on individual doctors or patients. The body of economic literature presented here should not be used to titrate care for the individual patient, although the embedded effectiveness data deserve attention even at the patient's bedside. Instead, these data should systematically inform policy decisions on how best to use society's resources to optimize clinical outcomes.

Second, the use of QALYs as a unit of effectiveness embodies a societal indifference to the recipient of health care benefits. A cost-effectiveness analysis using QALYs assumes that a QALY gained by an elderly patient with ischemic cardiomyopathy is identical to a QALY gained by a teenager with fulminant viral myocarditis; the goal then is to maximize QALYs across all patients. This indifference may or may not adequately capture societal preference; alternative approaches that emphasize certain age groups rather than others (eg, disability-adjusted life years) have been proposed but have not found wide acceptance in the United States. It follows that health economic analyses may clarify some important issues about the choices being considered, but must be overlaid with societal values and preferences while formulating health policy.

Several countries have established centers of excellence to rigorously evaluate the cost-effectiveness of new medical technology and systematically embedded these evaluations into drug approval (e.g., Ontario, Canada) or widespread adoption (e.g., the United Kingdom). On the other hand, the United States has thus far shied away from tying health care reimbursements to clinical outcomes. The recent health care reform bill explicitly forbids the newly formed Patient-Centered Outcomes Research Institute from the development or use of a cost-effectiveness threshold in considering which therapies it recommends for coverage or reimbursement.[4]

Experience has shown that Americans are capable of consuming vast quantities of health care resources, with no evidence of a limit to the potential demand for care. However, because there is a limited willingness to pay for such care, it is inevitable that some form of restraint on health care spending must be put in place. In the present highly polarized political environment, it may be the 1 thing that both ends of the political spectrum can agree on. A basic appreciation of the principles of health economics makes it evident that rationally adopted cost-containment measures do not need to equate to clinical compromise. Informed physicians, who have long viewed themselves as tireless advocates for their patients, must now play a leading role in steering American health care, slowly but surely, to a sustainable system that represents the best societal value for money.

REFERENCES

1. Health Data 2010: statistics and indicators. 2010. Available at: http://www.oecd.org/document/30/0,3746,en_2649_37407_12968734_1_1_1_37407,00.html. Accessed December 21, 2010.
2. CBO. The long-term budget outlook. Washington DC: Congressional Budget Office; 2007.
3. Roger VL, Go AS, Lloyd-Jones DM, et al. Heart disease and stroke statistics–2011 update: a report from the American Heart Association. Circulation 2011;123(4):e18–209.
4. Neumann PJ, Weinstein MC. Legislating against use of cost-effectiveness information. N Engl J Med 2010;363:1495–7.
5. Smith A. Qualms about QALYs. Lancet 1987;1: 1134–6.
6. Mark DB. Economics and cost effectiveness in cardiology. In: O'Rourke RA, Fuster V, Alexander RW,

editors. Hurst's the Heart Manual of Cardiology. 13th edition. NewYork: McGraw Hill; 2011. p. 2389–408.

7. Maisel AS, Krishnaswamy P, Nowak RM, et al. Rapid measurement of B-type natriuretic peptide in the emergency diagnosis of heart failure. N Engl J Med 2002;347:161–7.

8. Mueller C, Scholer A, Laule-Kilian K, et al. Use of B-type natriuretic peptide in the evaluation and management of acute dyspnea. N Engl J Med 2004;350:647–54.

9. Mueller C, Laule-Kilian K, Schindler C, et al. Cost-effectiveness of B-type natriuretic peptide testing in patients with acute dyspnea. Arch Intern Med 2006;166:1081–7.

10. Heidenreich PA, Gubens MA, Fonarow GC, et al. Cost-effectiveness of screening with B-type natri-uretic peptide to identify patients with reduced left ventricular ejection fraction. J Am Coll Cardiol 2004;43:1019–26.

11. Redfield MM, Rodeheffer RJ, Jacobsen SJ, et al. Plasma brain natriuretic peptide to detect preclinical ventricular systolic or diastolic dysfunction: a commu-nity-based study. Circulation 2004;109:3176–81.

12. Braunwald E. Expanding indications for beta-blockers in heart failure. N Engl J Med 2001;344:1711–2.

13. Effect of metoprolol CR/XL in chronic heart failure: Metoprolol CR/XL Randomised Intervention Trial in Congestive Heart Failure (MERIT-HF). Lancet 1999;353:2001–7.

14. Hjalmarson A, Goldstein S, Fagerberg B, et al. Effects of controlled-release metoprolol on total mortality, hospitalizations, and well-being in patients with heart failure: the Metoprolol CR/XL Randomized Intervention Trial in Congestive Heart Failure (MERIT-HF). MERIT-HF Study Group. JAMA 2000;283:1295–302.

15. Packer M, Bristow MR, Cohn JN, et al. The effect of carvedilol on morbidity and mortality in patients with chronic heart failure. U.S. Carvedilol Heart Failure Study Group. N Engl J Med 1996;334:1349–55.

16. The Cardiac Insufficiency Bisoprolol Study II (CIBIS-II): a randomised trial. Lancet 1999;353:9–13.

17. Packer M, Coats AJ, Fowler MB, et al. Effect of car-vedilol on survival in severe chronic heart failure. N Engl J Med 2001;344:1651–8.

18. Delea TE, Vera-Llonch M, Richner RE, et al. Cost effectiveness of carvedilol for heart failure. Am J Cardiol 1999;83:890–6.

19. Ekman M, Zethraeus N, Jonsson B. Cost effective-ness of bisoprolol in the treatment of chronic congestive heart failure in Sweden: analysis using data from the Cardiac Insufficiency Bisoprolol Study II trial. Pharmacoeconomics 2001;19:901–16.

20. Varney SA. A cost-effectiveness analysis of biso-prolol for heart failure. Eur J Heart Fail 2001;3:365–71.

21. Kazi D, Deswal A. Role and optimal dosing of angiotensin-converting enzyme inhibitors in heart failure. Cardiol Clin 2008;26:1–14, v.

22. Glick H, Cook J, Kinosian B, et al. Costs and effects of enalapril therapy in patients with symptomatic heart failure: an economic analysis of the Studies of Left Ventricular Dysfunction (SOLVD) Treatment Trial. J Card Fail 1995;1:371–80.

23. Effect of enalapril on survival in patients with reduced left ventricular ejection fractions and congestive heart failure. The SOLVD Investigators. N Engl J Med 1991;325:293–302.

24. Lee VC, Rhew DC, Dylan M, et al. Meta-analysis: angiotensin-receptor blockers in chronic heart failure and high-risk acute myocardial infarction. Ann Intern Med 2004;141:693–704.

25. Yusuf S, Pfeffer MA, Swedberg K, et al. Effects of candesartan in patients with chronic heart failure and preserved left-ventricular ejection fraction: the CHARM-Preserved Trial. Lancet 2003;362:777–81.

26. McMurray JJ, Andersson FL, Stewart S, et al. Resource utilization and costs in the Candesartan in Heart failure: Assessment of Reduction in Mortality and morbidity (CHARM) programme. Eur Heart J 2006;27:1447–58.

27. Taylor AL, Ziesche S, Yancy C, et al. Combination of isosorbide dinitrate and hydralazine in blacks with heart failure. N Engl J Med 2004;351:2049–57.

28. Angus DC, Linde-Zwirble WT, Tam SW, et al. Cost-effectiveness of fixed-dose combination of isosor-bide dinitrate and hydralazine therapy for blacks with heart failure. Circulation 2005;112:3745–53.

29. The effect of digoxin on mortality and morbidity in patients with heart failure. The Digitalis Investigation Group. N Engl J Med 1997;336:525–33.

30. Uretsky BF, Young JB, Shahidi FE, et al. Randomized study assessing the effect of digoxin withdrawal in patients with mild to moderate chronic congestive heart failure: results of the PROVED trial. PROVED Investigative Group. J Am Coll Cardiol 1993;22:955–62.

31. Packer M, Gheorghiade M, Young JB, et al. With-drawal of digoxin from patients with chronic heart failure treated with angiotensin-converting-enzyme inhibitors. RADIANCE Study. N Engl J Med 1993;329:1–7.

32. Ward RE, Gheorghiade M, Young JB, et al. Economic outcomes of withdrawal of digoxin therapy in adult patients with stable congestive heart failure. J Am Coll Cardiol 1995;26:93–101.

33. Eisenstein EL, Yusuf S, Bindal V, et al. What is the economic value of digoxin therapy in congestive heart failure patients? Results from the DIG trial. J Card Fail 2006;12:336–42.

34. Pitt B, Zannad F, Remme WJ, et al. The effect of spi-ronolactone on morbidity and mortality in patients with severe heart failure. Randomized Aldactone

Evaluation Study Investigators. N Engl J Med 1999; 341:709–17.

35. Glick HA, Orzol SM, Tooley JF, et al. Economic evaluation of the Randomized Aldactone Evaluation Study (RALES): treatment of patients with severe heart failure. Cardiovasc Drugs Ther 2002; 16:53–9.

36. Pitt B, Remme W, Zannad F, et al. Eplerenone, a selective aldosterone blocker, in patients with left ventricular dysfunction after myocardial infarction. N Engl J Med 2003;348:1309–21.

37. Weintraub WS, Zhang Z, Mahoney EM, et al. Cost-effectiveness of eplerenone compared with placebo in patients with myocardial infarction complicated by left ventricular dysfunction and heart failure. Circulation 2005;111:1106–13.

38. Zhang Z, Mahoney EM, Kolm P, et al. Cost effectiveness of eplerenone in patients with heart failure after acute myocardial infarction who were taking both ACE inhibitors and beta-blockers: subanalysis of the EPHESUS. Am J Cardiovasc Drugs 2010;10: 55–63.

39. Zannad F, McMurray JJ, Krum H, et al. Eplerenone in patients with systolic heart failure and mild symptoms. N Engl J Med 2011;364:11–21.

40. Juurlink DN, Mamdani MM, Lee DS, et al. Rates of hyperkalemia after publication of the Randomized Aldactone Evaluation Study. N Engl J Med 2004; 351:543–51.

41. Al-Khatib SM, Anstrom KJ, Eisenstein EL, et al. Clinical and economic implications of the Multicenter Automatic Defibrillator Implantation Trial-II. Ann Intern Med 2005;142:593–600.

42. Mark DB, Nelson CL, Anstrom KJ, et al. Cost-effectiveness of defibrillator therapy or amiodarone in chronic stable heart failure: results from the Sudden Cardiac Death in Heart Failure Trial (SCD-HeFT). Circulation 2006;114:135–42.

43. Sanders GD, Hlatky MA, Owens DK. Cost-effectiveness of implantable cardioverter-defibrillators. N Engl J Med 2005;353:1471–80.

44. Hohnloser SH, Kuck KH, Dorian P, et al. Prophylactic use of an implantable cardioverter-defibrillator after acute myocardial infarction. N Engl J Med 2004; 351:2481–8.

45. Bigger JT Jr. Prophylactic use of implanted cardiac defibrillators in patients at high risk for ventricular arrhythmias after coronary-artery bypass graft surgery. Coronary Artery Bypass Graft (CABG) Patch Trial Investigators. N Engl J Med 1997;337: 1569–75.

46. Cleland JG, Daubert JC, Erdmann E, et al. The effect of cardiac resynchronization on morbidity and mortality in heart failure. N Engl J Med 2005;352: 1539–49.

47. Cazeau S, Leclercq C, Lavergne T, et al. Effects of multisite biventricular pacing in patients with heart failure and intraventricular conduction delay. N Engl J Med 2001;344:873–80.

48. Bristow MR, Saxon LA, Boehmer J, et al. Cardiac-resynchronization therapy with or without an implantable defibrillator in advanced chronic heart failure. N Engl J Med 2004;350:2140–50.

49. Auricchio A, Stellbrink C, Sack S, et al. Long-term clinical effect of hemodynamically optimized cardiac resynchronization therapy in patients with heart failure and ventricular conduction delay. J Am Coll Cardiol 2002;39:2026–33.

50. Abraham WT, Young JB, Leon AR, et al. Effects of cardiac resynchronization on disease progression in patients with left ventricular systolic dysfunction, an indication for an implantable cardioverter-defibrillator, and mildly symptomatic chronic heart failure. Circulation 2004;110:2864–8.

51. Abraham WT, Fisher WG, Smith AL, et al. Cardiac resynchronization in chronic heart failure. N Engl J Med 2002;346:1845–53.

52. Young JB, Abraham WT, Smith AL, et al. Combined cardiac resynchronization and implantable cardioversion defibrillation in advanced chronic heart failure: the MIRACLE ICD Trial. JAMA 2003;289: 2685–94.

53. Higgins SL, Hummel JD, Niazi IK, et al. Cardiac resynchronization therapy for the treatment of heart failure in patients with intraventricular conduction delay and malignant ventricular tachyarrhythmias. J Am Coll Cardiol 2003;42:1454–9.

54. McAlister FA, Ezekowitz J, Hooton N, et al. Cardiac resynchronization therapy for patients with left ventricular systolic dysfunction: a systematic review. JAMA 2007;297:2502–14.

55. Kazi D, Hlatky M. The cost-effectiveness of cardiac resynchronization therapy. In: Abraham W, Baliga RB, editors. Cardiac resynchronization therapy in heart failure. Philadelphia (London): Lippincott Williams & Wilkins; 2009.

56. Calvert MJ, Freemantle N, Yao G, et al. Cost-effectiveness of cardiac resynchronization therapy: results from the CARE-HF trial. Eur Heart J 2005; 26:2681–8.

57. Nichol G, Kaul P, Huszti E, et al. Cost-effectiveness of cardiac resynchronization therapy in patients with symptomatic heart failure. Ann Intern Med 2004;141:343–51.

58. Feldman AM, de Lissovoy G, Bristow MR, et al. Cost effectiveness of cardiac resynchronization therapy in the Comparison of Medical Therapy, Pacing, and Defibrillation in Heart Failure (COMPANION) trial. J Am Coll Cardiol 2005;46: 2311–21.

59. Yao G, Freemantle N, Calvert MJ, et al. The long-term cost-effectiveness of cardiac resynchronization therapy with or without an implantable cardioverter-defibrillator. Eur Heart J 2007;28:42–51.

60. Fox M, Mealing S, Anderson R, et al. The clinical effectiveness and cost-effectiveness of cardiac re-synchronisation (biventricular pacing) for heart failure: systematic review and economic model. Health Technol Assess 2007. Available at: http://www.ncchta.org/fullmono/mon1147.pdf. Accessed January 1, 2008.

61. Hlatky MA. Cost effectiveness of cardiac resynchro-nization therapy. J Am Coll Cardiol 2005;46:2322–4.

62. Kazi D, Hlatky MA. (S)Ticker Shock: The Cost-Effectiveness of Cardiac Resynchronization Therapy With and Without an Implantable Defibrillator in Advanced Symptomatic Heart Failure. Am Coll Card 2008;51(10):A252.

63. Hunt SA, Haddad F. The changing face of heart transplantation. J Am Coll Cardiol 2008;52:587–98.

64. Cope JT, Kaza AK, Reade CC, et al. A cost compar-ison of heart transplantation versus alternative operations for cardiomyopathy. Ann Thorac Surg 2001;72:1298–305.

65. Digiorgi PL, Reel MS, Thornton B, et al. Heart trans-plant and left ventricular assist device costs. J Heart Lung Transplant 2005;24:200–4.

66. Miller LW, Nelson KE, Bostic RR, et al. Hospital costs for left ventricular assist devices for destination therapy: lower costs for implantation in the post-REMATCH era. J Heart Lung Transplant 2006;25:778–84.

67. Hernandez AF, Shea AM, Milano CA, et al. Long-term outcomes and costs of ventricular assist devices among Medicare beneficiaries. JAMA 2008;300:2398–406.

68. Rose EA, Gelijns AC, Moskowitz AJ, et al. Long-term use of a left ventricular assist device for end-stage heart failure. N Engl J Med 2001;345:1435–43.

69. Lietz K, Long JW, Kfoury AG, et al. Outcomes of left ventricular assist device implantation as desti-nation therapy in the post-REMATCH era: implica-tions for patient selection. Circulation 2007;116:497–505.

70. Wilson SR, Givertz MM, Stewart GC, et al. Ventric-ular assist devices the challenges of outpatient management. J Am Coll Cardiol 2009;54:1647–59.

71. Chan DC, Heidenreich PA, Weinstein MC, et al. Heart failure disease management programs: a cost-effectiveness analysis. Am Heart J 2008;155:332–8.

Index

Note: Page numbers of article titles are in **boldface** type.

heartfailure.theclinics.com

Printed and bound by CPI Group (UK) Ltd, Croydon, CR0 4YY

03/10/2024

01040346-0007